Transcending the Everyday Temptations of Overeating

Transcending the Everyday Temptations of Overeating

Vicki Arkens

iUniverse, Inc.

New York Lincoln Shanghai

Transcending the Everyday Temptations of Overeating

iUniverse books may be ordered through booksellers or by contacting:

iUniverse
2021 Pine Lake Road, Suite 100
Lincoln, NE 68512
www.iuniverse.com
1-800-Authors (1-800-288-4677)

The information, ideas, and suggestions in this book are not intended as a substitute for professional medical advice. Before following any suggestions contained in this book, consult your physician. Neither the author nor the publisher shall be liable or responsible for any loss or damage allegedly arising as a consequence of your use or application of any information or suggestions in this book.
The Scripture quotations contained herein are from the New Revised Standard Version Bible, copyright 1989 by the Division of Christian Education of the National Council of the Churches of Christ in the USA. Used by permission. All rights reserved.

ISBN-13: 978-0-595-41114-6 (pbk)
ISBN-13: 978-0-595-85471-4 (ebk)
ISBN-10: 0-595-41114-2 (pbk)
ISBN-10: 0-595-85471-0 (ebk)

Printed in the United States of America

For Bob
Your steadfast love and support made this possible

Contents

Part 3
The problem is: Willpower is no match for temptation
~ Strength will come ~

Part 4
The problem is: Self-monitoring increases self-involvement
~ *You can be set free* ~

Acknowledgments

First and foremost, I want to thank my husband, Robert Arkens, for his encouragement and invaluable advice on this project. You willingly shouldered the task of being the sole breadwinner so this book could be written. I also want to thank our three children—Caitlin, Landon, and Alice—for being a wonderful source of joy and inspiration to me. I'm deeply grateful to my parents, Donald and Elsie Waterman, for providing me, along with my brothers, Bob and Jim, with a love-filled home in which to grow up. And last, but not least, I'd like to thank my good friend, Deb Biechler, for editing assistance and for tireless listening throughout the seemingly endless revisions.

Introduction

Many years ago, I naively set myself to the task of finding a solution to the problem of overeating. I figured I should take control of my life and reinvigorate my motivation to eat well and lose weight. After selecting a diet and exercise program, I shored up my willpower and vowed to be vigilant in healthful eating behavior. I also believed that a religious discipline should be added to the effort. Armed with all of this, I thought I'd soon achieve permanent weight loss and be able to share my success story with others. I had no idea what I was in for.

There was so much I didn't know. I didn't know that my problem with overeating was going to intensify despite my attempts to take control. Nor did I anticipate that those wonderful times of high motivation were going to shrink. Willpower was going to weaken. The inner conflict was going to get the best of me. It seemed the harder I tried, the more I failed. I'm sure many of you know exactly what I'm talking about.

Eventually I realized there is a better way—a way of inner transformation. I know that sounds hazy as well as difficult. Yet it's far more real and reliable than willpower, and far easier than laborious self-monitoring. If we want to conquer any type of temptation, we must put forth our best effort. But, we also need the transforming power of God. From a new vantage point of spiritual living, we may transcend the everyday temptations that have become life-consuming problems.

The four-part format of this book will lead you through four spiritual principles that I believe are essential for positive self-change. This will culminate in the *Four Practices for Transcending Everyday Temptations* that can serve as a prayerful reminder of these effective and enduring principles. I feel certain the four practices will help you in your own problem with overeating. They will help you find freedom and self-mastery in all forms of temptation.

This book also offers an eating plan that is different from anything you may have encountered before. The *Four Habits for Normal Eating* are designed to diminish food cravings and naturally reduce food consumption. They will provide clarity and simplicity to your daily eating decisions. These habits will allow you to shift your attention from eating concerns to the greater goals of life.

I've interspersed my thoughts with passages from the book of Psalms and the book of Proverbs. Quotations from Psalms depict strong human emotion and spiritual longing. These ancient writers were not hesitant to address God directly as they reached out for help. Their religion was a firsthand, dynamic experience. I encourage you to follow their lead and experience God for yourself.

Sincerity is all you need to begin. Be willing to open yourself to the trustworthy love of God. The divine presence will restore you to wholeness and unveil a beautiful world of unimagined possibilities.

Part 1
There is a better way

Battle weary

We are very weary in the struggle with overeating. We wage this battle every day while discarded days of defeat mount up rapidly behind us. Yet each day seems like an eternity when resisting temptation.

We're tired of the familiar pattern in the quest for weight loss: pick yourself up from the last failed attempt, motivate to begin again, learn a new strategy, apply willpower, then keep on self-monitoring. Each new attempt meets with ever-diminishing success. Whether we have ten pounds to lose or one hundred, the pattern is the same.

Occasionally, we see someone emerge victorious, looking healthy and slim. We view them with a mixture of jealousy and admiration. Chances are we had some glory days too. Somehow, we managed to summon the enthusiasm and discipline to conquer the problem, at least temporarily. Yet, we know that trouble lies ahead for that new victor. There will be a gradual lessening of motivation, a growing tendency to cheat on the diet, ever-weakening willpower, and more excuses for not exercising.

We long to give up on the battle and turn our attention to other matters. But how can we? Do we give ourselves over to decreasing mobility, discomfort, and susceptibility to dis-ease—not to mention the depressing search for bigger clothes? Do we just smile and accept ourselves while we continue to abuse our bodies with too much food?

Why is it that there are countless numbers of competent people, who are disciplined in so many ways, yet totally at the mercy of this temptation? This one, very basic aspect of life has become a never-ending, losing battle.

We search through stacks of diet books for answers. We listen to talk shows for a bit of sage advice. We scan the covers of magazines for clues. People step forward to tell us their stories, and there are many suggestions that make sense. A few years ago, I read an opinion page in a national magazine, written by a man who had solved his overeating problem. Every time he wanted to reach for food, he sat down until his feelings of anxiety subsided. He concluded that, if everyone did that, there'd be far fewer weight problems. I wish that were so. He's lucky he has just one reason he overeats; and to his credit, he found a way to stop his pattern. Many overeaters are not so fortunate. We must fight the battle on many different fronts.

We're helplessly confused in the complexity of the problem. We overeat for a variety of reasons. As soon as we subdue one reason, another rises up and tackles us from behind. We eat to calm ourselves in emotional stress. We celebrate with food. We eat to relieve boredom. We eat when we feel insecure. We love to taste, chew, and warm ourselves with food. We examine ourselves and search out the reasons for our behavior. It's apparent that eating has become the catchall response to any kind of discomfort, need, or longing.

Food surrounds us constantly, keeping us in a perpetual state of conflict. It's exhausting to referee these clashing desires. We desperately want freedom from the prison of this inner struggle. We long for some reliable measure of self-mastery amidst temptation. Yet, the power to succeed has completely vanished.

In the numbness of confusion and weakness, we realize that only God can help us. We know we can't fight this on our own anymore. We've stretched the limits of our human capacity to change. We feel powerless. We've been knocked down one too many times, and we can't stand up. With fervent longing, we turn to God. And he is there. We are not alone and we need God desperately.

Tragedy and temptation make us realize that we need God. In crashing waves of tragedy and dangerous whirlpools of temptation, we reach for the hand of God.

O Lord, all my longing is known to you;
my sighing is not hidden from you.
My heart throbs, my strength fails me;
as for the light of my eyes—it also has gone from me.

Psalm 38:9–10

Lean on God

The time has come to stop everything and rest a while with God. Sit down next to him and lean upon the everlasting arms. You need to be alone with God. It is good to rest with him when you can't even think to pray, or when you can't take a step forward. You don't need to do anything or say anything—just rest.

God is very close to you. He is a magnificent presence in the universe yet also very near to each one of us. The creator is loving and merciful, as well as powerful and just. We are not alone in the universe, nor are we alone inside our own minds. He is our intimate companion.

We can trust God's love. He loves each one of us with a great affection. We are precious to him. His love nourishes us and heals our inner wounds. Seek comfort and reassurance from the divine heart. We can depend upon him with simple, childlike trust. He understands us and he knows our frailties.

We may also trust his great power. We can feel secure that, with God, we can overcome all problems. With God there is always a way. In him, there is victory no matter what happens. There are fresh perspectives and unforeseen answers. With God, we can feel safe despite the outward circumstances of life. We may trust his promises and abundance.

We need to experience God, and that experience is very personal. He can be our perfect parent, closest friend, adored teacher, or beloved sovereign. Some may prefer the image of Divine Mother. I refer to God as "Father" most often, because the word evokes in me a trusting intimacy as well as an image of benevolent power. My use of male pronouns reveals that preference. The name you choose for God should fit what feels right to you and what you need.

> *He makes me lie down in green pastures;*
> *he leads me beside still waters;*
> *he restores my soul.*
>
> Psalm 23:2–3a

Lay down your burdens

After a time of rest, don't be afraid to tell God anything that comes to mind. Lay down your burdens. Share your confusion. Tell him that you don't know where else to turn. Acknowledge that you feel overwhelmed. Divulge your feelings of defeat. Your regrets about overeating may be numerous: I feel out of control ... I dislike what has happened to my body ... I've dulled my mind and robbed my energy ... I don't trust myself anymore ... I'm sick and tired of my ways.

As you are opening yourself to God, you may find that painful feelings about other things will surface. It is well known that emotional pain causes us to be more vulnerable to the temptation of overeating. We try to soothe the inner pain with the balm of food. Name your feelings as best you can. Confess, or acknowledge that you feel afraid, angry, worried, guilty, ashamed, bitter, or jealous.

Feel free to confess anything you feel bad about. Acknowledge your mistakes, errors of judgment, inattention, insensitivity, and anything else you might regret. Don't prejudge your confessions by reserving confession only for blatant acts of selfishness or resistance to God. Slowly unwind the tightened knot of false security. Release your grip on what troubles you. Release your painful feelings to God. Release your fears and failures into God's care. Empty out so that there is room for God's healing love to come in.

Confession calms when we're full of conflict and defeat. It actually feels good to confess when we're lacking the desire to move forward, when we feel powerless, and when we're confused. Confession has a restful quality. In confession, we let down our guard of self-defense. Just be honest. You no longer have to put up a front. You're simply stating what is, without explanation or embellishment. It is an honest statement of what you know down deep. It's what you can see when all pretenses are gone.

> *Turn to me and be gracious to me,*
> *for I am lonely and afflicted.*
> *Relieve the troubles of my heart, and bring me out of my distress.*
> *Consider my affliction and my trouble,*
> *and forgive all my sins.*

Psalm 25:16–18

We've depended on food

In the calm clarity of confession, we begin to see that we depend upon food for many reasons. We reach for food to fill an unnamed emptiness, when we need to feel whole and secure. We search out food to calm down, when we need to unwind and relax. We use food to break out of boredom, when we need a spark to stimulate. We turn to food for fun, when we want some pleasure out of life. Food is our comforter and our protector. Food is our tranquilizer. Food is our energizer. Food is our entertainer.

As we look back on how we've used food, a pattern begins to take shape. We use food to provide ourselves with:

- Security
- Relaxation
- Stimulation
- Pleasure

We depend on food for fundamental feelings of security, relaxation, stimulation, and pleasure. Food, a basic source of satisfaction, is used to provide basic feelings of well-being. If this is true, perhaps this idea can be taken one step further. We can match these rather modern, psychological words with the following, ancient words of higher spiritual meaning:

- Love

- Peace

- Hope

- Joy

Notice how love matches security. Peace easily corresponds with relaxation. Hope coincides with stimulation. Joy fits well with pleasure. Much has been written about the emotional hunger for love, as being a primary cause of overeating. That wonderful insight gets to the heart of the human need for security and self-esteem. Yet we see there are other hungers we are trying to satisfy. We may search for a sublime sense of inner peace. We may long for a light of hope in the midst of discouragement. We may want more out of life, even the promise of joy.

Love, peace, hope, and joy—are these what we seek when we engage in temptation of any kind? Are they elevated feelings, perhaps spiritual emotions? Can we sum them up in one word—happiness? If so, then we come to understand that we're searching for happiness when we overeat. We've depended on food, rather than God, in our search for happiness.

Happy are those who find wisdom, and those who get understanding,
... Her ways are ways of pleasantness, and all her paths are peace.

She is a tree of life to those who lay hold of her;
those who hold her fast are called happy.

Proverbs 3:13, 17–18

Indulgence of a natural tendency

We might define temptation as an indulgence of a natural tendency in the search for happiness. Often, people use the word addiction when the indulgence feels like it is completely beyond their control. The classic, religious definition of temptation involves the choosing of the way of self over the way of God. Keep that in the back of your mind, but for now, I will focus on the first definition.

Indulgence, in the case of overeating, is the consumption of any type of food well beyond the need of nourishment. Often, this involves overeating foods that are unnaturally attractive. Healthful consumption of food, however, allows for normal taste gratification and normal hunger satisfaction.

It goes without saying that eating is a natural tendency. There are strong physical reasons underlying the urge to eat and overeat. They will be examined in more detail later. These physical reasons seem to be stronger in some people than others, which partially accounts for why some people overeat and some do not. Many of us have a natural tendency to overeat, and modern life encourages those tendencies. Happiness is the goal, and the natural tendency is the means.

As a father has compassion for his children,
so the Lord has compassion for those who fear him.
For he knows how we were made; he remembers that we are dust.

Psalm 103:13–14

Gripping happiness

In the search for happiness, we've inadvertently veered into the realm of this temptation. Once we're in, we try so hard to keep a grip on happiness with it. We use food not only to find, but also to control, our own happiness. And control is a dominant feature of modern life.

Look at what our culture is telling us. We've been taught to believe in ourselves and to depend on ourselves as the way to conquer any problem. We believe we should be self-sufficient and self-directed. It tells us to create our own reality of individual happiness. We hardly notice our secular thinking because it is an integral part of our culture.

We even practice spiritual disciplines as a means of controlling our happiness. Occasionally I receive flyers in the mail that tell me I can attract good things to my life through doing a special set of disciplines. There is little said about humility and self-surrender. Genuine religion promises happiness—but not through the ways of the world.

In earlier times, life was hard and more uncertain. You felt blessed if you saw your children become adults and if you had enough food on the table. Agricultural societies were completely dependent upon the weather. Hunger was a very real possibility and ordinary diseases easily brought death. The common people of old were not so much interested in happiness as in simple human dignity. They knew by hard experience that people couldn't expect to control every aspect of life.

The more civilization advances, the more security we seek. We have unemployment compensation, safety regulations, and modern medicine. We strive to be fully insured and cushioned from hardships. By the standards of the developing world, we are the secure rich with disposable incomes, spacious homes, and several cars. At the same time that we have greater control over the basics of life, we face new temptations, continuous distractions, a faster pace, unceasing change, and endless details. No wonder modern society has an "obesity epidemic." Amidst the unique stresses of modern life, food is a readily available source of basic satisfaction and security.

Of course, we know that overeating is an unreliable means of controlling personal happiness. The pleasure of eating a frosted donut, the momentary stimulation of chocolate candy, the relaxing effect of crunching tortilla chips, the feelings of security from a large hamburger and fries—are all fleeting. Despite our advanced and discriminating knowledge about food, we return to it repeatedly for good feelings and the easing of bad feelings.

Overeaters use food to escape even the smallest sufferings of daily life. We may feel trapped by an unpleasant circumstance. We dull uncomfortable emotions with the distraction of a snack. We continually try to escape the assorted pains of life. When I found myself inventing numerous excuses to indulge, I realized I was refusing to suffer. Temptation becomes both a shortcut to happiness and an escape from the usual irritations of life.

Through frequent and heavy indulgence, the temptation loses its ability to provide even a temporary refuge or a paltry happiness. The way of temptation promises much but delivers little. We return to it again and again, yet satisfaction remains elusive, moving further beyond reach. In our attempts to control our own happiness, we've been robbed of it. We start out trying to control life with this temptation, but the temptation ends up controlling us.

Sadly, we have become compulsive about eating. If we're around food, we've lost the ability to say no. The sight of food draws us like a magnet. Eating has become the center of life. It is the glue that holds life together. We've used food to escape the difficulties of life, and now eating has become a prison. We have become dependent on the temptation.

> *Sometimes there is a way that seems to be right,*
> *but in the end it is the way to death.*

Proverbs 16:25

Depend on God

Sooner or later, we all face something that is our undoing. It demonstrates to us that we cannot be strong by ourselves. We need to depend upon a higher power. We must transfer our dependence on things, on activities, on other people, or on substances of abuse, to a sublime dependence on God. Some of us meet up with a temptation that incapacitates us. Some of us face tragedy that immobilizes us. A startling disappointment may stop us in our tracks. We all have an Achilles' heel. I look around at people I know, and I wonder how they manage so well without God. What is their secret? Perhaps it's a coping strategy. People look fine on the outside, but there are private burdens and vulnerabilities that likely lurk below the surface.

When we face that which brings us to our knees, we become humble. No longer are we in charge. In the humility of this realization of our own powerlessness, the barriers go down and we turn to God. Humility before God is a cleansing state of vulnerability and openness. Humility makes us receptive to the help

God has always been offering. We confess that we need God in order to change.

It can come as a tremendous relief to surrender the sense of self-sufficiency after experiencing greater and greater conflict in the attempt to keep life under our control. Confession of dependence releases us from the rigidity of false fronts and the supports of futile resolutions. A softness of emotion develops gradually when we shift from self-reliance to dependence on God. Honesty comes more easily after we've laid down the sword and shield of self-defense. This admission of dependence can be disconcerting. One of the paradoxes of religion is that, through dependence on God, we become whole.

When we depend on God for happiness, we trust that we will receive. With him, we find comfort and inner healing. His personal presence brings love, wisdom, power, and goodness. When we trust God's abundance, we find that we don't need to turn to food so often to get ourselves through the day. We can stop trying to manipulate our own happiness. His promises are real. Place your happiness in God's hands, trusting rather than manipulating. Have faith in his nurturance and compassion. Trust God for the fundamental aspect of happiness—a sense of security and love.

How precious is your steadfast love, O God!
All people may take refuge in the shadow of your wings.
They feast on the abundance of your house,
and you give them drink from the river of your delights.
For with you is the fountain of life;
in your light we see light.

Psalm 36:7–9

Restoration of self

The transfer of dependence from food to God can be made more difficult by a wounded sense of self. Many people carry persistent feelings of shame, unworthiness, helplessness, inferiority, or incompleteness. You may have a fear of abandonment that makes you feel helpless. Your parents may not have cared for you very well or loved you unconditionally. There may be persistent hurts from the tragedies of life such as the death of a loved one. You may have experienced a loss that affects your feeling of wholeness.

All this results in emotional pain that is carried deep within us. If these wounds happened in childhood or have persisted for a long time, there can be conditions of numbness or paralysis of will, making it difficult to respond normally to other people or to life. The pain may come from something that happened long ago, or it may be going on right now. Walls of self-defense can be terribly hard to break down. Some of us may need counseling. A fearful or wounded animal has a hard time trusting the person who is trying to help.

As I mentioned earlier, painful feelings can create a greater susceptibility to overeating or any type of compulsive behavior. Food is used as a balm to soothe or hide the pain inside. Eating becomes the place of reference and security. It has become the primary means of comfort. Some of us may truly be eating for love.

Those whose self-respect has been wounded especially need assurance of God's trustworthy presence. Allow the wounds to be healed by God's comforting love. You need to feel cared for. Experience the security that comes from his love. You need to know that you are his precious child and that you have a unique place in his world. You can take on a new identity with God as your father. Let down your defenses and accept his reliable care and steadfast affection.

The Lord is near to the brokenhearted,
and saves the crushed in spirit.

Psalm 34:18

◆   ◆   ◆

Pause often, to rest a while with God. The struggle with this temptation has been long and frustrating, so keep enjoying the rest.

If you find it hard to depend on God, you may have some confusion about God that is blocking it. Children sometimes grow up with a frightening image of a stern God that interferes with a trusting relationship. Some people hold an image of God that is very distant and uninvolved. Allow yourself a little time to believe that God is interested in you and that he is loving, comforting, and protecting. God is close to you and he cares for you. He chose you before you even began to look for him. God has high hopes for you, yet he knows that you have a long way to go. He is patient and kind. He goes with you through the good times and the bad. You are never alone.

But you, O Lord, are a God merciful and gracious,
slow to anger and abounding in steadfast love
and faithfulness.

Psalm 86:15

Part 2
Higher desires can flourish

After a renewing period (of rest and full dependence upon God,) the desires of life will begin to stir. But don't stand up just yet. Stay close to God and share these desires with him.

Confide in God

Within the security of God's love, you can be entirely honest. Begin now to lay out your desires before God in prayer. Some of these desires may be needs, and others may be wants. Some may be aspirations but others far less than noble. Don't sort through your desires for appropriateness. Just lay them all out. It will be quite a jumble, but at least it's an honest jumble.

Talk to God as if you're talking to a friend. He knows you very well. Nothing you say can surprise him or shock him. No desire is too insignificant to share with God, and no longing is too embarrassing to acknowledge. You might uncover many different layers of desire within yourself, ranging from base to high. Often we have glorified aspirations, mixed with lower desires.

As you pray, other thoughts may intrude. Reminders, plans, and ideas often break in on prayer. Each one demands your immediate attention, but they all can wait. Simply offer them to God along with your prayers. Fears and irritations that were lurking in the corners during confession may suddenly appear. Sometimes an unrecognized desire struggles to make itself known within an intruding thought. If you can, name that desire as you lay all these thoughts before God. Don't be harsh with yourself. Be patient, like God. You are the master of your mind. Gently bring your mind back to prayer.

Ask also for wisdom. So often, God answers our prayers with a valuable insight. This is especially true if you are seeking guidance about a particular problem. You may be entirely confused about what needs to be done or even what you want. Sometimes you have a vague idea of something you need to pray about, but you can't phrase it. In that case, say, "Please, speak to me of this." You may be holding a problem that is shot through with emotion, making it difficult to sort through. God helps us in the process of discernment. His guidance is always gentle.

Prayer is different from the repeating of self-affirmations in which one might say, "I *can* overcome my habit of overeating." It is different because you are seeking help from a greater power. Self-affirmations draw only upon human willpower. In the attitude of prayer, you are acknowledging your need of God and trusting God as you share your longings.

Find a time and a place to pray that really works for you. If you don't like to sit still, you could try walking and praying. Walking can help the mind stay focused. If you habitually awaken in the night, that wakeful period can be an excellent time to pray. If you have trouble staying awake, there's nothing wrong with praying while you sip early morning coffee.

Prayer does not have to take a long time, and you don't have to pray about everything all at once. Just pray the desires that come easily into your mind. Words are not even necessary. A sincere attitude of seeking help from God is all that is really needed.

Have patience and be persistent in prayer. Earlier in my life, when prayer was irregular and sometimes long neglected, I noticed that a fervent request took a couple of days to realize an answer. It was as if the path from God to me was overgrown with brambles through lack of use. I imagined that God had to bush-whack his way through to reach me, thus creating a time lag. As I prayed more regularly, the time between request and answer became considerably less. Our persistence in prayer does not change the mind of God, but it does improve our receptivity.

But it is for you, O Lord, that I wait;
it is you, O Lord my God, who will answer.

Psalm 38:15

Conflicting desires

Through our healthy human desires, we initiate the forward movement of life. It is perplexing when these desires seem to run out of steam and sometimes die altogether. If you've started diets with strong resolve that soon fades, you know how frustrating this problem with desire can be. It is a problem of vital concern in the struggle with any type of stubborn temptation.

I'm sure you've noticed that a potent desire to eat healthfully and lose weight comes along only sporadically. It seems that a powerful desire just happens once in a while—we can't create it or control it. Many of us have completed at least one temporarily successful diet. When it comes time to diet again, the enthusiasm of the first time is hard to get back. We wish for health and fitness all the time, but wishing doesn't mean we're willing to work for it. The problem is, our desire for self-improvement is fluctuating and unstable.

Why is genuine desire for self-improvement so sporadic? We humans always seem to be in conflict with our higher and lower natures. Unfortunately, the lower nature is so stubborn. It is very difficult to extricate yourself from the grip of a lower desire once it has taken hold, especially if it is a natural tendency. Once the thought of overeating enters your mind, it becomes a slippery slope to the action itself.

Does this seem familiar? The thought of food enters your mind. Your attention becomes riveted to the thought. The longer the thought sticks in your mind, the more you are tempted. Good excuses for indulgence pop into your mind. You turn to fight the temptation with reasons why you shouldn't. If that doesn't work, you bring out an arsenal of affirmations. You say to yourself: I like knowing I'm burning fat for energy … I *can* coexist with tempting food … Food is not so important to me anymore … I'm more powerful than food. Alas, you can't find a foothold upon which to stand. The desire for food wipes out your higher inclinations, and you can hardly remember why you want to lose weight. The desire for change, and the miserable effects of the habit, all fade. You can't get a grip. Your mind is a confusing tangle except for the thought of eating. You may as well give in.

So much of life is wasted in this recurring battle. As soon as we find ourselves arguing with temptation, the likelihood of victory is small. Immediate gratification always seems to win out over the argument for deferred gratification. We can't just substitute a higher desire for a lower desire. We can't battle a lower desire by trying to summon power from a higher desire. We're in constant conflict, at war in ourselves. It's a prison of inner conflict.

Years of this kind of conflict weaken us to the point where we lack the freedom to choose the higher desire. Lack of freedom is the defining characteristic when someone is compulsive about food. We frequently hear people say, "Oh, don't put that candy dish near me!"—and for good reason. The thought of the candy will dominate that person's mind while they sit there. Eating is no longer a choice. It's compulsory.

So how do we escape this perpetual inner conflict? If arguing with temptation doesn't work, what will? Can we successfully strengthen our higher desires? Before I talk about the effective answer to these questions, let's look at motives.

> *Save me, O God,*
> *for the waters have come up to my neck.*
> *I sink in deep mire, where there is no foothold ...*

Psalm 69:1–2a

Motives can be improved

We've been taught to strengthen our higher desires through awakening and energizing the underlying motivation. Weight loss experts try to whip us into a frenzy of enthusiasm. They shout, "Get motivated! You can do it! Lose ten pounds before summer! Be the thin person you've always wanted to be!" All this cheerleading lights a fire in us, but the stoked up desire soon burns out.

We actually have two main desires. One desire is to eat normally—to stop overeating. The other desire is to lose weight. These two desires are distinct, but easily confused. The desire to lose weight dominates over the desire to eat normally. Eating normally is nice, but what we desperately want is to lose weight. If we lose weight, yet still have abnormal eating patterns, we feel successful. If we start to eat normally, yet are still overweight, we feel like failures.

The motives underlying the desire for losing weight can range from base to high. Some motives can be quite prideful. We want to lose weight so we can be fit and trim at the class reunion, so we can show off on the beach, so we can wear that fabulous outfit and be the envy of everyone at the party. The appeal to vanity doesn't permanently strengthen our higher desires. We need to be aware that pride can undermine our determination in this battle with overeating. Pride is spiritually weakening. In the same way, the more we grow spiritually, the less power prideful motives have in producing change within us.

We benefit from naming and nurturing the higher motives for conquering overeating. As we let go of the old prideful motives, we can reach for something new and better. We need motives that are less selfish. We need spiritually infused motivations. Perhaps create a visualization in which you name some of the higher motives for eating normally and losing weight. For example:

- I want to feel energetic. When I don't overeat, I feel clear, light, and clean inside. I want to feel healthy and strong. Losing the burden of excess body fat would feel liberating.

- I want to be as beautiful as is naturally possible. My imperfect yet unique beauty is a reflection of the beauty of creation. I also know that people who love me will appreciate seeing me happier, healthier, and shining with natural beauty.

- I want to be ready and able to help. When my body isn't clogged with food, I feel more capable of lending a hand. I'm ready for service. I'm not distracted by the desire for food or slowed by feelings of fullness.

- I want to think more clearly. My mind operates better when I'm not overloaded with excess food to digest. I'm better able to make decisions and carry them out. When my mind is clear, my spiritual capacity is enhanced.

- I want to respect my body as a temple for the divine presence. Good habits and healthful consumption of food honor the life God has given me.

Even after idealistic motives like these are named and encouraged, a true desire to eat normally and lose weight can be frustratingly sporadic. The question remains: how *do* we strengthen our higher desires? Improving our motives is admirable, but it is not the highest, most effective answer.

All one's ways may be pure in one's own eyes,
but the Lord weighs the spirit.

Proverbs 16:2

Let go

I started out by saying we need to lay out all our desires. Now it's time to give them to God and let go of them. Offer your prayers to God and make sure to release them into his care. Give *all* your desires to God for safekeeping. Entrust your longings to him and allow God to hold them for you. In letting go, we are surrendering our desires to God.

Chronically conflicting desires must both be offered. So often, we pray for help and healing while still clutching the temptation. You may be surprised to find that the desire to indulge food cravings is still lodged in your mind. You prayed for and let go of the desire to eat normally, but the conflicting desire has been overlooked and is still deeply rooted in your mind. Since the desire to overeat is a major problem in your life, make sure to give this tenacious desire to God. You may be subconsciously holding onto it, keeping it for yourself. Sometimes we try to hide things from God or even from ourselves.

When we give the tempting desire to God, we trust that, in some way, satisfaction will come. We can give our food desires to God and trust that we will experience food satisfaction. All things are possible with God so long as we accept that we will receive in the way God provides. We need to understand that he magnifies what is natural and honorable in the tempting desire. He will provide for our wants as well as our needs, in his time and in his way.

It's likely you will find other tempting desires lodged in the corners of your mind. These also should be given to God. We especially need to stop harboring desires that are compelling mind preoccupations. These are pet thoughts that chronically block the letting-go process. Temptations of the mind need to be surrendered to God. They weaken and may even degrade us. The sanctuary of the mind should not shelter the continual replaying of obsessive thoughts.

It's hard to let go of a precious desire. It's as if we have a pleasing possession that we would never want to just drop by the wayside. We can surrender the possession more readily if we trust that the precious desire will be remembered and in some way preserved. When we need to deal with the desire again, we may find that the desire isn't quite so compelling after we have taken a break from it. It may have even transformed into something that has spiritual value while in the care of God. God preserves what is real in all that we have surrendered.

In the spiritual life, there is an emptying and a filling. Relinquish anything that keeps your mind busy and distracted. Do the best you can to make room for the presence of God—even if it is just a bit of cleared space. Then, take the vital second step. Let God into your mind.

Trust in him at all times, O people;
pour out your heart before him ...

Psalm 62:8a

Let God in

God has always been with you, but now deliberately open yourself to receive his presence. Let God into your conscious mind. When you do this, you are still you, but your mind is filled with God. I like to think that my *self* inhabits the center of my body, and my mind is a dwelling place for God. When you allow God into your mind, the mind is illuminated by his presence. You become God conscious and spirit filled.

When God is your constant companion, you are sharing your inner life with him. This intimate sharing is more than confiding a few secrets to a friend. It is like sharing a room with that friend, and that room is the mind. Think *with* God rather than *about* God. You're never alone inside your mind.

There have been long periods of time when I wasn't able to offer my whole mind to God. I literally wasn't willing to share everything with him. If that is a problem for you as well, clear a space in the center of your mind for God. Then allow God into that center. If you do that, you'll find the center growing until at last you are able to allow God into your whole mind. Every dark corner of the mind will be enlightened by his presence.

Life will start to change when you do this. The awareness of the divine presence is worth any price. Just the willingness to share your inner life with God can begin this transformation. The desire for spiritual growth will embrace you. You'll start to see the world differently. You'll gain a proper perspective on the temptations that have dogged you. Your higher desires will begin to open and grow.

For God alone
my soul waits in silence ...

Psalm 62:1a

Higher desires thrive

When we let go and let God in, our higher desires are nurtured and the lower desires recede. Thus, the problem of the fluctuating strength of our higher desires is solved. Temptations lose power when they are in the hands of God. The conflict between the higher nature and the lower nature becomes easier to handle. Our desires are adjusted and a new perspective emerges.

Consciousness of the divine presence is unifying. We are no longer divided and at war within ourselves. With God, we experience oneness and wholeness. When the mind is a sanctuary for God, his presence brings peace.

This process of letting go and letting God in is like doing the will of God. We surrender our desires to him and then let God's will into our lives. Doing God's will is a natural outcome when we are one with him. When we are sharing our inner life with God, we are, in effect, doing God's will. Therefore, it can be said that our higher desires flourish within the will of God.

> *O Lord, you will hear the desire of the meek;*
> *you will strengthen their heart,*
> *you will incline your ear*

Psalm 10:17

The will of God

The will of God can be a difficult concept for modern people. We are very suspicious of anything that seems to take away personal control and liberty. The will of God may also be laden with unhappy connotations. It may have been offered as a way of explaining something incomprehensible, such as the sudden death of a loved one. Sometimes it has been used to keep people confined to a tradition. Words like surrender and submission come into play and make us even more apprehensive.

In contrast to our trepidations, the will of God is expansive and infinitely creative. It's not a prescribed set of activities. There are endless possibilities within the will of God. When one chooses the will of God, one is participating in all that is true, beautiful, and good. The will of God is gracious and trustworthy. Most people acknowledge God as the creator and upholder of all that we know of life and reality. It only stands to reason that God's way embraces all that is found to be in harmony with greater life and deeper reality. God's will is the way that leads to a better life and true happiness.

The will of God is actually freeing. It feels like a burden has been lifted when we realize that all we have to do today is God's will. We no longer feel trapped by our own ways of dealing with life. We are no longer imprisoned by selfish desires and priorities. God's will puts everything into manageable perspective. This can come as a relief to modern people who are burdened with confusing and complex decisions. We don't have to feel bound by the expectations of other people and the slavish attention to the endless details of modern life.

Holding the desire to do God's will in your mind is less complicated than a series of rules. His will is the steady focus. There is no longer a need to be carefully mindful of disciplines, procedures, plans, and behavior. God knows the perfect path for you. Doing the will of God is the full and complete answer. The wholehearted desire to do God's will is the answer that solves all problems.

Doing the will of God is the great mystery of religious life. How can it be that, in surrendering our desires to his will, our higher desires are made manifest? Why is it that, when we lay down our own will and accept God's will for our own, we find true freedom? Other religious mysteries pale by comparison to the transformation that takes place when we lay down our will for God's.

The will of God allows us to move forward one step at a time. It doesn't push us faster than we are able to go. Our higher desires are strengthened and stabilized. The desire to

cleanse our selves of temptation is nurtured through our dedication to the will of God. We're on our way to becoming balanced and unified.

> *Commit your way to the Lord;*
> *trust in him, and he will act.*

Psalm 37:5

Beware of debilitating emotions

We've begun to experience the peace that living in God's presence brings. But beware that painful emotions will try to creep
back in. Fearful or angry thoughts attempt to sneak back in as
we go about our day. Embarrassments and irritations may rush
in during a moment of weakness or when we awaken in the
night. We've confessed these feelings to God. We also must
refuse to allow them to reenter.

Emotions play a large part in overeating; however, I've mentioned emotions only briefly with regard to confession. It is well
known that the stress of emotions may cause us to lapse into
overeating. Stress has a huge effect on food consumption, causing some people to eat more and some people to eat less. Overeaters may harbor anger at people who have pushed them to
lose weight. The stress of this anger may sabotage your current
efforts to change.

I've noticed that some people are more prone to fear and others more susceptible to anger. These are habitual emotional
responses to the problems of life. Fear serves a practical purpose
to keep us out of danger, but most of our fear reactions are
unhealthy. For those of us who easily become fearful, it takes
some convincing to realize we don't have to live with the pain of

fear. Anger can be cleansing (initially)—the first step in healthy self-assertion and rightful indignation. Chronic anger, however, rapidly devolves into belligerence and blaming. Anger might be even harder to let go of than fear. While fear is entirely painful, we get a perverse satisfaction out of being angry. Fear and anger weaken us and poison any hope of a happy life.

We don't have to be emotionless, however. We can experience natural, downside emotions that are not contaminated with fear or anger. For example, I experience sadness and sorrow as cleansing emotions. I run into big trouble when I twist these pure emotions with fear or anger. A mixture of sadness and anger begets bitterness. Sorrow brewed with fear induces feelings of shame or chronic guilt. Allow your pure emotions and welcome the tears when they come.

If you ever feel like you can't get control of your mind, give your whole mind to God. There are times when your mind can be stuck in fear or obsessive thinking. Even when your mind is unmanageable, you can control your will enough to ask God to take over. If you ever feel that your own mind is your enemy, seek emergency help. Ask for the mind of God to take over completely, at least for a period of time. Psychological counseling and medicine may also assist us. Do not confuse your conscience with God. The conscience can be harsh, but the leading of God is always gentle. Emotional healing is inner healing. We are made inwardly whole when the presence and love of God are within us.

Emotionally laden problems are very difficult solve. Giving the problem to God and taking in his presence help us get a proper perspective on even our most terrifying problems. It is so important to get our problems out of the mind and let God adjust our distorted thinking. We need the perspective and understanding of divine wisdom. We need to trust that God will help us see more clearly, and we need to know that he is with us in our struggles. When it is time to think about the problem again, think of it in God's presence. Think *with* him. You do not have to handle anything alone. With God, there is always a way. He will illuminate a clear path through the tangles and thorns of every problem.

God is more than willing to heal us of fear and anger, but we need to release our grip on them as well. Every effort we make to let go of them will be met with an addition of divine power. We have work to do alongside God in the healing process. Do not hold in your mind those things that induce you to feel fearful or angry. Don't keep a graveyard of bad memories and failures. Welcome, instead, the convictions of love and confidence. Rather than thinking about your regrets, problems, and fears, keep placing them in God's hands. Welcome his love and be filled with his peace. Seek God's presence and rededicate yourself to his will.

> *Refrain from anger, and forsake wrath.*
> *Do not fret—it leads only to evil.*
>
> Psalm 37:8

◆   ◆   ◆

It is here that prayer of supplication ends, with a dedication to God's will. The will of God steadies and fortifies our higher desires. Life in the will of God brings peace from inner conflict. Living with God makes us whole and unified. The guidance of his will leads to discernment and wisdom. Surrendering to God opens the door to real freedom. The presence of God makes life simple and beautiful.

Now we face the world, and there are challenges ahead. Stand up with God and prepare to step forward with him.

Your decrees are wonderful; therefore my soul keeps them.
The unfolding of your words gives light;
it imparts understanding to the simple.

Psalm 119:129–130

Part 3
Strength will come

After a time of commitment to God's will and presence, prayer comes to an end. We refocus on our surroundings. The duties of life beckon.

Stand up with God

When you prepare to leave your time of prayer, stand up with God. Don't leave him behind. You've invited God into the main room of your mind; now keep that consciousness of his presence. Too often we say, "Amen," then get up all by ourselves. We finish praying, only to face the world alone, armed with shaky resolutions. We cut off God's help before we even get started.

When you try to stand up again after prayer, that is when you may realize how wobbly you still are. It takes a while for a sense of strength to develop. Strength develops best as you keep that presence of God with you as you go about your day. Remember, you don't have to face the world alone. He will help you feel steady and capable of meeting the challenges of life. You may rely on the Spirit to guide you through the difficulties and decisions that lie ahead.

It's unsettling to move abruptly from the stillness of prayer to the demands of life and the duties that await us. So, take a bit of time to prepare. Soon we will come face to face with the problem we've prayed about. Food is everywhere we turn: donuts at the office, candy displays in the checkout line, and fast-food commercials on television. The pressure is on. Consequently, as we stand to meet the challenges of the day, there is a feeling of apprehension. We've stumbled so many times before. Is this time going to be any different? Can we really launch a renewed effort to resist temptation?

> *Make me to know your ways, O Lord; teach me your paths.*
> *Lead me in your truth, and teach me,*
> *for you are the God of my salvation ...*

Psalm 25:4–5a

The limitations of willpower

To meet the challenge of resisting temptation, we've been taught to assert our willpower. Motivational speakers exhort us to develop a can-do attitude. They urge us to visualize ourselves being successful. They tell us, "You can change your life. Exert the power within you! Give yourself positive affirmations. You can be who you want to be, and you can do what you want to do!"

Overeaters know all too well that willpower is not reliable. We know how many times we've steeled our resolve before a food occasion, only to utterly collapse when the occasion arrives.

We know that we can feel strong and resolute one minute, but as soon as someone offers us a gooey chocolate chip cookie, the positive self-talk is forgotten. We know how weak we are around food. It seems as if we've become weaker with each refurbished resolution. Through repeated failure, our vigor and hopefulness are fading. Summoning willpower—again—becomes a meaningless exercise. We know we need strength for the effort, but where is this strength going to come from?

We've tried to shore up our willpower by thinking positively. We look around and see that some people use the technique of positive thinking, without any religious perspective, and it seems to work for them. They are strong-willed and highly self-motivated. They exemplify the high ideals of humanism. We compare ourselves to those ideals and wonder what's wrong. Why are we not able to self-generate that can-do attitude? Why is our willpower so inadequate?

Even the strongest among us might eventually meet up with something in life that we cannot overcome through our own strength of will. Life is bound to hand us a challenge that defies positive thinking and willpower. Overeating is certainly one of those challenges. The energy to solve it requires more than the human capacity for change. The more we try to overcome it, the more victory eludes us. Willpower actually seems to diminish with each new assault on the problem.

I've noticed that spiritually growing people often feel that sense of weakness quite acutely. The conflict between the higher nature and the lower nature becomes more noticeable. The old motives for self-change don't energize us. There is a disconcerting awareness that the self has exhausted its own power.

For so long I didn't understand this, and I fought against the weaknesses in myself. As I grew older, the weaknesses became more threatening. My own self-assertion became increasingly unable to overcome my inherent weaknesses. We need to make the complete switch from self-reliance to God-reliance. The more you advance spiritually, the more dependent you become upon God. The higher you climb, the more you need the power of the Spirit.

> *Seek the Lord, and his strength;*
> *seek his presence continually.*

Psalm 105:4

The time of transition

There is a time of transition in spiritual growth that can be very difficult. It is the time between your first sincere faith reach to God and when you consistently allow him into your life. That transition is the time of our lives when we've ceased to rely solely on human strengths and worldly motivations, yet we haven't thoroughly grasped God's hand.

Nature provides many analogies of transitions. When a spaceship is launched from earth, the time of pushing through the earth's atmosphere is turbulent. When the ship reaches space, all is peace. When a woman is giving birth, there is a time called transition, which is the most harrowing. It is the time just before the final stage of the birthing process.

This zone of transition makes us very unsure of ourselves. That is why spiritually growing people feel vulnerable. We feel divided between the ways of the world and the ways of the spiritual realm. Unfortunately, many of us have spent much of our lives in the transition. We've acknowledged our need for spiritual growth and lifted up our hands in faith, but we haven't left the old ways

behind. We haven't entirely entered into the new life of the Spirit.
How do we do this?

To you, O lord, I lift up my soul.
O my God, in you I trust …

Psalm 25:1–2a

Release the sails

We've raised the mast; now fully release the sails of faith. We've
already used our faith in a limited way. Begin to make full use of
its potential. Faith is the mysterious method of spiritual life. Faith
has been given to us from God, as a means of moving forward and
ascending upward into the liberated life of the Spirit. We've recognized our dependence on God for life and identity. We've
opened ourselves to his intimate presence. Now, let us make full
use of his gift of faith.

Living faith is dynamic confidence in God. It is life changing.
Faith begins with an attitude of sincerity or earnestness, even
childlike trust. Eventually, our faith is strong enough to believe
that God will lead us through all the difficulties and uncertain-
ties of life. We trust that he will show the way. We know we will
be guided as we move along the path of life.

Some may view the reliance on faith as a dangerous thing.
Indeed, faith can be misused if you refuse to face facts. Faith
must not deny the realities of God's creation. Faith will not fail
you so long as you have an open mind to divine truth. Faith
must be based upon a dedication to God's will. We must be
morally and intellectually honest. Honesty and openness to
truth go hand in hand with effective faith.

Faith liberates the potentials within you. Even if your faith seems very weak, hoist it up anyway. The more you do this, the sturdier it will become. Faith has been given to us to use. You have the gift of faith at your command. Your faith enables you to cross over into a new and better life. Be persistent. Muster your faith at every turn. Keep your mind open to divine truth and your faith sail raised.

When we release the sails of faith, the unfurled sails catch the breath of God. The wind of the Spirit fills us and strengthens us. The Spirit sheds the light of truth and the power to live life to the fullest. This is salvation from selfish desire—salvation from the temptations of modern life. This is spiritual transformation.

> *Trust in the Lord with all your heart,*
> *and do not rely on your own insight.*
> *In all your ways acknowledge him,*
> *and he will make straight your paths.*

Proverbs 3:5–6

Faith and effort

In the strength of this renewal by the Spirit, we can proceed with power to do our part to conquer temptation. Human effort is essential. Life is arduous, so we may as well learn to relish the struggle. The chick must peck its way out of the shell, and the butterfly must labor to open its untried wings. By contrast, the way of temptation is laced with indolence and impatience. But the way of God calls forth our best effort.

The way of God also summons our faith. We enter the spiritual life by faith, and we progress by this same gift of faith. As we wend our way through life, we can achieve an artful balance between human effort and the gift of faith. Some people expect God to do everything for them. Others forget God and try to make their way through life solely on their own power. In the end, victory crowns the efforts of all who rely upon faith.

God can effectively guide the person whose life is in motion. The pilot can steer the boat as it glides. Through our faith, the Spirit uplifts and magnifies all our efforts in the solving of life's problems. Do the best you can, but remember to deploy your faith.

When troubles come, you and God can manage them—together. No doubt, there will be troubles today. There will be emotional discomforts and unexpected pitfalls. Be assured that no matter what happens, God is beside you. Remember, you don't have to figure everything out on your own. You don't have to face life's problems alone. Allow God to lead you through the temptations and decisions that arise each day.

What is the effort needed here? Overeaters must find and execute a set of dependable habits for self-control. We need to make decisions ahead of time to prepare for the onslaught of temptation. Then we must carry out those decisions, through all the instantaneous choices that confront us in daily life.

The human mind plans the way,
but the Lord directs the steps.

Proverbs 16:9

A plan for self-control

Overeaters need a reliable way to navigate through the sea of food choices. We must make decisions about when, what, and how much to eat. Most of us need to learn a strategy or plan for eating. This plan should provide a foundation upon which to practice increasing self-control.

There are many plans to choose from. People who do not have to battle this temptation may shake their heads in wonder at all the diet books overflowing the shelves of bookstores. The different approaches can be difficult to learn and are often conflicting. The need for a nutritious variety of food makes the overeater's problem a seemingly hopeless tangle. We can't abstain from food as an alcoholic abstains from alcohol or a smoker abstains from cigarettes. Food is necessary to life, and there is natural satisfaction in eating.

I wanted a plan that did not deny natural body needs. Methods of self-control should work with nature, not against it. I didn't want to place unnatural restrictions upon my body. Feelings of self-denial easily cause discouragement and rebellious attitudes. Deprivation gives rise to the development of abnormal eating patterns. Under those conditions, we become even more obsessive and compulsive about food.

In addition, I desired a plan that would be simple to remember, convenient, satisfying, and healthful. I wanted to follow this plan yet be able to eat the evening family meal. Eventually I realized that I yearned to find an eating plan that would help me actually feel like a normal eater rather than an overeater. I wanted this plan to be adaptable to periods of noticeable weight loss. I often wondered, "Am I asking too much?"

Before proceeding to Part Four, I will present the eating plan I call the *Four Habits for Normal Eating.* I created it for myself, but I sincerely hope it will help many overeaters. Before launching into this eating plan, I have some further comments to make regarding the necessity for spiritual strength. Once we settle on a plan for self-control, there are problems of human weakness that continue to assail us.

> *Like a city breached, without walls,*
> *is one who lacks self-control.*

Proverbs 25:28

Mortal imperfection

No matter how simple the plan, making your way through the eating day is still fraught with unexpected challenges and sudden lapses. Probably the most devastating is when you've successfully followed your plan all day; then, at the very end, an inexplicable moment of weakness hits and you start searching the cupboards. In the face of such failure, the overeater must not lose hope. Some days will be confusing and difficult. Yet, on other days, everything seems to come together. We can't expect to be perfect, but we can keep trying to make increasingly better choices. No one said it was going to be entirely smooth sailing. There will be stormy days and sudden squalls.

Despite the best-laid plans, food temptations can still catch you off guard. Without warning, the thought of eating something delicious overtakes your mind, and you can't set it aside. The thought comes with flowers and a cheery smile. It says to you, "A bit of food could liven you up … Go ahead, celebrate a little … Loosen up and enjoy life … You deserve to take a break … You've been under a lot of stress." The excuses for eating are endless. We succumb far more often than we like to admit.

The classic religious struggle is between the way of temptation and the way of God—the way of evil versus the way of good. Some people believe that God deliberately tempts us in order to test our obedience to his will. Others believe that an evil power has a hand in even the small temptations of life. For many believers, both of these attitudes have given way to a prominent belief that God created a world in which we have freedom to exercise our free will. Our imperfection guarantees that we will have to battle with the temptations that arise out of our natural tendencies and our human selfishness if we are to succeed. Happily, the struggle and growing allegiance to God's way make us strong and thoroughly loyal.

I don't think it's helpful to castigate yourself for disobeying God when you transgress your eating plan. You don't want to create a feeling of separation from God over such a small matter. It is true that you've settled on a plan with God through the insight gained in prayer. We're sure that God wants us to be healthy and free of this temptation. But God also knows we are imperfect and that we take two steps forward and one step back as we progress. He is not shocked and angered by our predictable, mortal failings.

In my younger days, I tried vowing to God that I would follow my eating plan perfectly, and I managed to do so—for three whole weeks. Then, something threw me off track and I had a big relapse. So there I was, mad at myself for cheating on my plan and feeling estranged from God. The parental nature of God probably smiled and caught me as I fell. He knows that the making of vows, which we're not mature enough to keep, is bound to fail. He knows our weaknesses, but he wants us to get back up and keep on trying. Failure is part of the learning process. We fail as we move forward.

Don't waste time and energy by feeling guilty about transgressing your eating plan. Arrogant willfulness and stubborn resistance to God are the major problems that threaten your spiritual life. Overeating pales by comparison to those temptations. Confess your failing, pick yourself up, and dust yourself off. Renew your dedication to God's will by opening your mind to his presence. Then recommit yourself to your eating plan.

> *I will study the way that is blameless.*
> *When shall I attain it?*

Psalm 101:2a

Self-deception

Human frailty is not the only cause of failure. We must also be aware of the subtleties of self-deception. Without realizing what is happening, I start telling myself lies, and I believe them. I tell myself, "A little relaxation of my plan won't hurt … I can stop when I want to … It's OK to go this far … I'm going to test myself … I think I need to remember what it was like before … I'm stronger now, so I'll be able to handle it." Self-deception creeps in to undermine our hard-fought decisions. We fall back into old ways so easily and before we know what we are doing.

Self-deception quietly invades after we have begun to feel a sense of God-bestowed power. We easily forget the source as we glory in our newfound strength. Self-deception gives us a false sense of self-sufficiency. It makes us think we are powerful on our own. We start thinking we can engage in a limited form of temptation when we really cannot—and should not. Eventually, the flow of strength from God runs dry because we haven't maintained the connection with God.

We must guard against those deceptive feelings of self-sufficiency. We need to remember that we are dependent upon God. It is so important to remain humble. Don't let subtle pride gain a foothold. It is the Spirit, in conjunction with our faith, that bestows true strength. We must be honest with ourselves and remember that this power is not our own. Giving thanks is a powerful antidote to pride. Remember how far you've come. Give thanks for the power you've received.

> *Pride goes before destruction,*
> *and a haughty spirit before a fall.*
>
> Proverbs 16:18

Beware of doubt and discouragement

Lastly, a few words need to be said about doubt and discouragement. Beware of doubt that pulls down the sails of faith. At first, the chains of doubt are more familiar and comfortable than newfound freedom in faith. We question whether we really can withstand the assaults of temptation. We wonder if the breath of God really will fill the sails. We pull back in doubt about the effectiveness of this entire, spiritual approach to life. If this happens, give your doubts to God, as you've given everything else. Make room for a renewed infusion of God's presence and his gift of faith.

Discouragement also pulls down those sails of faith, so take note when you feel it coming on. Discouragement can actually be a daily habit. Discouragement lures us to turn back and to give up. Notice your breathing and posture. A collapsed feeling in the body can bring on a collapse in the sails of faith. Do you overreact to minor setbacks in your day? Does disappointment bring you to a standstill? Do you give up easily in the face of challenges and difficulty? Do you become overwhelmed by the demands of life? If so, stand up and take a deep breath. Refuse to harbor discouraging thoughts and give them at once to God. Summon your faith and be filled with the Spirit.

The root of discouragement is fear, a lack of courage. I've spoken about the dangers of fear before, but it is worth noting again. Fear oppresses your faith. So many of us lead lives made small by shrinking fear and stunted by paralyzing anxiety. We must take a stand against fear. Weed it out before it takes hold of your mind and give it to God in exchange for the powerful convictions of love and confidence. Take command of your mind and, with God, unfurl the sails of faith once more.

Do not let loyalty and faithfulness forsake you;
bind them around your neck,
write them on the tablet of your heart.

Proverbs 3:3

◆　　　◆　　　◆

Sometimes we fall so hard we need to rest for quite a while before we have the strength to get up. Be patient with yourself. Allow yourself a healing time of stillness with God. And when you are ready, begin again.

Through faith, you will be lifted up into a new way of living. From this vantage point of spiritual living, the conflicts of life will no longer threaten to defeat you. The problems that seemed insurmountable may be conquered. You will experience genuine power for living. This new experience provides the assurance that transcending temptation is possible.

Be of good courage,
and he shall strengthen your heart,
all ye that hope in the Lord.

Psalm 31:24 (KJV)

Four Habits for Normal Eating

Overeaters know the techniques of weight loss, but we know very little about normal eating. Pounds are lost during times of high motivation, but because we don't understand how to eat normally, the pounds quickly return. Years of dieting have driven us even further away from the ability to make natural eating decisions. We've become slaves to our food cravings, insensitive to stomach fullness, confused about what to eat, and subject to stress-induced eating.

The good news is: overeaters can learn to eat normally. Presented here are four practical habits to recover normal eating behavior. If you form these habits, food cravings will diminish and food consumption will naturally decrease. In addition, food decisions will simplify, and stress-induced eating will subside. In short, you will actually begin to feel like a normal eater.

The *Four Habits for Normal Eating* are convenient, easy to remember, satisfying, and natural. There are no special recipes to prepare and no detailed menus to follow. This is a reliable and flexible plan for all eating situations. It will help you steer safely and surely through the eating day.

This plan did not suddenly occur to me one day. It evolved from experiences and observations I made over a long period of time. As I tried different eating plans, I began to keep track of the underlying physical reasons why I overate. I realized that I wanted to design a plan that would help to alleviate these causes. One of the first causes I noticed was what I call the taste-thirst connection. So this is where I will begin.

The taste-thirst connection to food cravings

Overeaters have terrible troubles with taste. The pleasure of taste lures us to food and keeps us fascinated. We overeat, in part, because we love the taste of certain types of food. Sometimes we enjoy these foods so much we say we're addicted to them. For many people, chocolate is the food that feels addicting. For others it is salty snack food. Still others are drawn to an array of tantalizing foods.

The snack food industry exploits that incredible longing for taste. It produces an endless variety of colorfully packaged treats created by combinations of sugar, salt, fat, and chemicals. Convenience foods make it too easy to indulge our taste buds all day long. We try various ways to suppress the appetite; but for those who are lured and fascinated by taste, the urge to eat is still there. Some overeaters overindulge only at mealtimes. Yet, many of us love to snack with abandon between meals.

By contrast, thin people drink beverages between meals. I noticed this when I was at a shopping mall one day. A thin young mother passed me, trying to console her fussy pre-schooler. I overheard her say, "Let's go get something to drink." It occurred to me that if the young mother had been overweight I might have heard, "Let's go get something to eat." That is certainly what I would have said. I would have gone in search of a tasty snack food. After that, it seemed like everywhere I looked,

I saw thin people depending on all manner of sugary beverages to get them through the day. They did not concern themselves with the calorie count or sugar content of the beverage. At parties, the thin people would sit back, content with a regular soda or glass of wine. Heavier people would cling to a sugar-free soda, while glancing furtively at the snack table.

I also noticed that thirst played an important role in how much food I consumed. If I was thirsty, I ate more. Often, I didn't even know I was thirsty. I would misinterpret my thirst as the desire for food. Food was the answer to all discomfort, even the discomfort of thirst.

As I observed these things, I wondered if the typical overeater has a stronger than normal taste urge, in addition to difficulty in discerning thirst. Do these two problems work together to increase the desire to eat?

I began to believe that thirst, combined with the desire for taste, becomes a powerful physical inducement to overeat. It's possible this is what brings about many strong food cravings. Taste and thirst both originate in the mouth, not the stomach. It's as if the desire for taste is intensified by thirst. Even the experience of binge eating seemed strangely like drinking. The rapid and continuous consumption of food is strongly suggestive of gulping water when very thirsty.

Based on these subjective observations, I decided to allow, if not encourage, myself to rely upon a wide variety of beverages. In doing this, I hoped to take a giant step toward satisfying, or at least calming, that mischievous taste-thirst urge. I was also simply copying what I observed normal eaters doing.

Sugar: substance of ill repute

My decision to drink all sorts of beverages brought up a big problem. The sugar content of beverages is highly controversial. Many believe that sugar is a major factor in the so-called obesity epidemic. Experts say refined sugar is just not healthful and that it makes us vulnerable to various diseases. Conventional wisdom holds that sugar causes a surge of energy with a corresponding energy crash. Many overeaters crave sugar, and sugar has become the enemy.

On the other hand, the desire for sugar is entirely natural. Breast milk is sweet, encouraging the baby to keep drinking for energy and growth. Thirst, plus the natural attraction to sweet flavor, was vital to our early development. It's no wonder we love sugar.

Despite the warnings, I decided to take my cue from babies and drink sweet beverages between meals for energy and taste satisfaction. I hoped this would satisfy my sugar cravings and even calm my salty food cravings. I wanted those attractions to frosted donuts and chocolate chip cookies to fade as I trained my taste buds to seek and expect sweet beverages. I also wanted to make beverage decisions based upon my own reactions. I did not experience that dreaded energy crash from a sugar high. I found that a sugared beverage tides me over a rough spot in the day, actually giving me energy rather than destroying my energy.

I had to keep encouraging myself to drink sweet beverages because I was hesitant to "spend calories" in this way. Veteran dieters who know their way around calorie charts know that a sugared beverage can wreak havoc with their daily calorie total. In my dieting days, I always skipped beverages in favor of a snack. Thus, I wasn't worried that I was going to go overboard with this decision. Perhaps the problems with sugar, as with most things, can be traced to excessive use. A six- and-one-half-ounce bottle of cola was the standard size when soft drinks were first marketed. Now, soft drinks are served in twelve-ounce cans, twenty-ounce bottles, or even larger sizes.

What's wrong with soft drinks?

Like many overeaters, I used to drink diet cola, as a strategy for calorie reduction. I stopped doing that in light of my new decision. Normal eaters sip sweetened beverages not only for taste satisfaction, but also for sugar energy between meals. When an overeater drinks an artificially sweetened drink, they are getting less taste satisfaction from the beverage and no energy lift. That fact alone can make one vulnerable to snacking. Why confuse your body by drinking something that pretends to be sweet, but has no energy value?

Following this line of thought, I began to drink the sugared version of the diet cola I used to drink. I felt somewhat guilty about it though. After all, soft drinks are one of the junk foods that health-conscious people shouldn't indulge. Nevertheless, I did happily drink it for quite a while with no weight gain or apparent health problems. But, there was something wrong about it.

I compulsively chose soda over other, more natural and nutritious beverages. If given a chance, drinks like apple juice are more effective in satisfying that taste urge which comes around with such persistence. I started to suspect that soda interfered with thirst quenching and even taste satisfaction. It actually seemed to dull or numb the taste buds. Even though soda was less effective, I kept returning to it throughout the day. I'd look past the attractive juices and consistently grab the bottle of cola.

For me, cola is the real culprit. It wasn't soda so much as it was cola I was compulsive about. I have no statistics to cite, but I observed that overeaters are more likely to depend upon diet cola than just any diet soda. If I eliminate cola as a choice, my compulsion about soda goes way down. When I look at a fruit-flavored or white soda alongside a glass of juice, the juice has a fighting chance to be chosen.

As I was mulling over the soda dilemma, a friend of mine said that, when she drinks a favorite cola soft drink, it makes her crave things like French fries rather than more healthful food. That struck a chord with me. I've come to believe that soft drinks support our attraction to junk foods. Soda and salty snack food are strongly linked. One seems to foster the attraction of the other. After you numb your taste buds and introduce the unnatural flavor of cola, your taste urge vigorously emerges, especially for salty snack food. If we could remove soft drinks and salty snack food from the American diet, it's possible many children would lose their excess weight and be able to enjoy a natural childhood, free of encumbering pounds.

Another problem with soft drinks pertains to the amount we are physically able to drink. We can drink much more soda at one time than juice. The carbonation in the soda makes it easy to quaff a twelve-ounce can. We use carbonation to settle the stomach, but that also allows us to drink more than would be natural. A typical breakfast juice glass is five ounces by comparison. That small size probably came about because large amounts of juice can cause stomach discomfort. Many people can't drink a lot of juice without suffering ill effects. That discomfort will remind you not to drink so much at one time.

Because of these problems with soft drinks, I had to qualify my decision to drink freely of beverages. Now I drink juice beverages and water between meals. I had a hard time giving up cola because it had been beneficial to my original efforts to rely on beverages between meals. At first, I still drank my favorite cola but in significantly lower amounts. I drank it only at certain times and made sure to reserve plenty of time to enjoy the juices and water that are truly beneficial. Now I drink it only occasionally. I'll return to the issue of soft drinks later because I know other overeaters will struggle with this as I did.

Sweet, tart, and salty beverages

There are many types of juice beverages to choose from. Fortunately, many beverages are readily available and more combinations are being developed almost as fast as new snack foods are produced. Convenience stores sell a generous assortment of beverages, which is a good trend. It's nice to see all the juices, bottled attractively, alongside the usual soft drinks.

For ease of recall, I divide beverages into five categories. The first three categories are juice beverages that correspond to the taste types of sweet, tart, and salty. Then I list the protein and water beverages. Examples are given for each category as follows:

Sweet:	Apple juice and blends, grape juice, apricot nectar, hot cider
Tart:	Orange juice, grapefruit juice, lemonade, cranberry cocktail
Salty:	Tomato juice, vegetable juice
Protein:	Milk, soymilk, yogurt beverage
Water:	Ice water, herbal tea, sparkling water, (coffee, tea)

A juice beverage may include everything from 100 percent juice down to the fruit-flavored drinks that contain very little juice. For nutrition, real juice is the better choice. Juice is also superior in flavor to a fruit-flavored drink. That may not seem so initially, but the more you drink juice the less appealing the juice drink will be. I don't exclude even those beverages that have no juice at all, so long as they are similar in flavor to real juice. For example, a popular powder mix beverage may have no juice in it, but at least it attempts to imitate juice. I'll choose these drinks if there are no other juice choices. I do not include the sugar-free juice drinks because the taste is artificial and it provides no energy lift. If you're used to natural juices, the sugar-free juice drinks can be quite unpleasant. The natural sweet of sugar truly enhances the fruit flavors that I try to emphasize.

At first, I had to remind myself to drink juice beverages. I easily skip them or forget about them because they don't create a compulsive reaction in me as cola does. If I start skipping those juices, my mind drifts over to some of the old taste desires for chocolate or salty snack food between meals. On the other hand, if I make sure to have a sweet or tart juice beverage between meals, I stay in touch with the more natural taste sensation of fruit. When I'm pressed for time, I'll quickly drink a five-ounce glass of juice to keep training myself to expect fruit flavors. If you keep up the habit of drinking sweet and tart juices, your taste buds will respond favorably to them.

Little changes can make a big difference in your liking for juice beverages. For example, I rarely chose apple juice because it tasted densely sweet to me. Then I realized that whenever I drank juice I never put ice into the glass. When I started doing that, my enjoyment of apple juice greatly increased. The ice lightens up the heavy flavor of the apple juice. Ice can also thin the beverage, making it less sugary, which may be preferable to many people. Juices with pureed fruit in them are thicker and smoother in consistency, which many people enjoy. They are also more nutritious, with the added benefits of whole fruit. Orange juice with pulp is a good choice, with no added expense.

You may discover that you like certain types of beverages at predictable times of day. I usually like a sweet beverage such as apple juice in the morning. Tart beverages such as orange juice or lemonade go well in the afternoon with some black tea. I save salty beverages like tomato juice for late afternoon.

Drinking tomato juice helps reduce cravings for salty snack food. In addition, when I drink a salty vegetable juice before supper, it prevents me from overeating for salt satisfaction at suppertime. People who habitually crave salt can at least be reassured that their salt needs are being met by drinking a mildly salty vegetable juice. Any taste desire is intensified by thirst, so keep drinking water in addition to the salty beverage. Salt cravers might even try drinking a sweet or tart beverage, to redirect their habitual craving for salt.

I recommend establishing a beverage path through the day. A beverage path helps you navigate more easily through the eating day. It reminds you of the possibilities for beverages between meals. You can bring in some of the protein beverages and water beverages that are listed. For example, in the morning I usually have coffee, cranberry apple tea, and apricot nectar. In the afternoon, I typically drink orange juice, black tea, and later, tomato juice before supper. In the evening I have milk and peppermint tea. I intersperse these beverages with cups of water.

I like to think of this beverage path as a type of therapy. I find I'm more compliant if I consider my beverages to be treatment for a disorder. If a doctor had ordered me to drink six ounces of a sweet juice in the morning, six ounces of a tart juice in the afternoon and six ounces of a salty vegetable juice before supper, I would have been even more cooperative. A beverage path is therapeutic in the sense that it helps to alleviate one of the physical causes of overeating—the strong desire for taste which is amplified by thirst. Juice beverages, in particular, will train taste desires and mildly satisfy the taste-thirst urge between meals.

I mentioned milk as part of my beverage path in the evening. Protein beverages like milk may be considered as a beverage or as a food to be consumed at mealtimes. I drink milk at least twice a day, once as food during breakfast and once as an evening beverage. I do not include the fully sweetened milk beverages, like chocolate milk, as a free choice beverage in this list. A pint of chocolate milk or strawberry milk, as sold in convenience stores, is very tasty and can be gulped down in seconds. Hot chocolate can't go down so fast, but it is still fully sweetened. I noticed that I consistently chose these sweetened milks over the juice beverages, so I knew they had to be taken out of my beverage list. Fully sweetened milk beverages are placed in a different category that will be explained later.

Water beverages include ice water, herbal tea, sparkling water, as well as the caffeinated beverages like coffee and tea. I put beverages containing caffeine in parentheses as a note of caution. Too much caffeine can make you feel out of control, less capable of reading your own body signals, and thirsty. Those effects can work together to sabotage better drinking and eating habits. Therefore, be careful with caffeinated beverages.

Sparkling water, sometimes called seltzer or club soda, is an acceptable alternative to the usual soft drinks. It does, however, have some of the same problems as other carbonated beverages, such as numbing the taste buds. Nevertheless, it can be useful to relieve stomach discomfort and will help you transition away from the usual soft drinks.

It's a good idea to alternate water with juice beverages. That way your consumption of sugar doesn't go beyond moderate to excessive. Six ounces of water seems to be the typical amount that people can drink at one time if they're not noticeably thirsty. If you find yourself hanging around the kitchen with nothing to do but get into trouble with the snack cupboard, take a drink of water. It's easy to quaff a small cup of water while you're standing by the faucet.

When you have the time to sit and enjoy a water beverage, find ways to make water more appealing. Choose an attractive glass for ice water. Enjoy the gentle clink-clink of ice cubes against the glass. Perhaps squeeze a bit of lemon in your water as they do in restaurants to make water look and taste more interesting. Brew herbal tea in a favorite large mug with a comfortable handle.

It's wonderful that we can buy bottles of water almost everywhere we go these days. There was a time when it was hard to find water if you were traveling. If the water fountain in the corner wasn't working very well, you were forced to buy a soft drink. Plain water is the source of life, and it's important to stay in touch with that.

Water: cooling, warming, settling, soothing

The drinking of water is very beneficial to the overeater in some obvious and some not so obvious ways. First, it quenches thirst. Second, it can be consumed to warm or cool the body. Third, it can soothe and settle the digestive system after eating.

It helps to know when your need for water is greatest. You may be thirsty upon waking up in the morning and not even know it. So, drink some water before your morning coffee. Don't forget to drink after physical exertion. That's when you'll really be able to take in a lot of water. If you know very well you need water, but you're having trouble making yourself drink enough, try drinking a lightly sugared beverage instead. It amazed me how quickly I could drink a glass of watered down lemonade after I'd been dawdling over a bottle of water. It's as if sugar uncovers the real underlying thirst.

When you need warming up, drink some hot herbal tea. Drinking a hot beverage can counteract the tendency to eat for warmth. Seeking warmth is another one of the physical reasons we overeat. Living as I do, in a colder climate, I found I sought out food when I felt chilly. Just as birds eat to maintain body temperature, we humans try to stoke our internal fires with food. The raw veggies and fruits that please us in the summer hold less attraction when the temperatures drop. For warmth, we're drawn to starches and high fat foods.

Make the effort to find a blend of herbal tea that you like. Some are made from a mint leaf. Some are spicy or cinnamon flavored. I particularly like ones that are fruity in flavor. Even if you think you don't like herbal tea, find one that is acceptable and try to get used to it. When you make a large mug of tea, you only need to drink a small amount. Warming your hands on a mug of tea is half the enjoyment.

On the other hand, water can be consumed when you need cooling off, both physically and emotionally. Stress produces a sensation of internal heat that cold water can alleviate. I noticed that I would get a hot feeling in the stomach when I was upset. Not surprisingly, I turned to food, like ice cream, to soothe and cool that hot feeling in the gut. I also used my favorite cola for that purpose. After I realized what I was doing, I found that cold water meets that need to cool down just as effectively. Now, I sip cold water during the internal heat of stress, as well as during the summer heat.

Cold water has another important use for the overeater. I learned to sip cold water after a meal to destimulate the taste buds and to settle and soothe the digestive track. Try this and take time to feel the cold water as it slides down the esophagus and into the stomach. I'll mention this repeatedly because it is very helpful in ending meals. Overeaters need to know how to end a meal before they get too full. I used to drink water before meals in the attempt to fill up so I wouldn't eat too much. Now, I save ice water to end the meal with the soothing sensation of cool water.

Problems with hunger and fullness

At the same time that overeaters are highly sensitive to the pleasure of taste, we also have an appalling lack of sensitivity to feelings of stomach fullness. The painfully stuffed feeling doesn't register until it is far too late. Normal feelings of fullness bring on a secure, contented feeling, but being stuffed is miserable. Do we habitually ignore our fullness signals? Are the signs of fullness simply too weak in overeaters? Do we refuse to remember how miserable it is to feel stuffed as we keep repeating the same mistake?

Normal eaters eat when they are hungry and stop eating when they are full. They are not tempted to snack between meals because they still feel satisfied from the previous meal. Conversely, they are hungry at regular mealtimes because they haven't been snacking. No matter how delicious a mealtime food is, they stop eating when their body signals it's time to stop.

Normal eaters have a strong sense of fullness. In some cases, they literally can't eat another bite even after they have consumed a moderate amount of food. I've watched someone who has never gained an ounce look longingly at a piece of pumpkin pie after dinner, but the sense of fullness was so strong that even lifting her fork for a taste seemed painful. Some normal eaters simply can't eat beyond a certain point, almost feeling ill at the thought of more food.

I've tried to monitor the fullness sensation in myself. It registers very faintly after a moderate amount of food, but if I keep eating, it goes away entirely. Curiously, I sometimes felt a bloating of the lips or face rather than the stomach signal that I expected. Sometimes I would feel a closure at the back of the mouth or a weakness in the limbs. The gut discomfort of fullness comes at least a half hour after I've stopped eating, too late to be of help. If I eat to the point of satisfaction, I will feel full a half an hour later. If I eat to the point of fullness, I will feel painfully stuffed later. How I wish that stuffed feeling would come before it's too late!

I realized something else that was disturbing. The painfully stuffed feeling is alleviated by—starting to eat again! A normal eater would never think of beginning to eat again if they felt uncomfortably full. But the overeater turns to food in the face of any discomfort, even the discomfort brought on by feeling stuffed. The more I overeat a meal, the more likely it is that I will start snacking.

It's a health disaster when someone has a strong taste urge coupled with a weak fullness signal. In addition, when the pain of fullness kicks in, it can be alleviated with more eating. Science can tell us more about the physical symptoms of fullness and why some people have such a hard time feeling them. If obesity runs in families, perhaps this weak fullness signal, plus the misreading of taste-thirst cues, is due, in part, to heredity. When I was toying around with these ideas, our family had two guinea pigs as pets. One continually ran to the water bottle for a drink during the day. The other returned repeatedly to the food dish. I'm sure I don't need to tell you which guinea pig was overweight. Was it a genetic predisposition that made one guinea pig crave water and the other food?

I like the non-diet idea of eating anything so long as you only eat when you're hungry and stop eating when you're full. This sensible idea is simple and straightforward. Unfortunately, I just couldn't make it work for me. I felt almost panicky as I tried to be mindful of hunger and fullness. I knew I was going to need a bit more help in order to make that idea work.

Easy-to-manage foods

While contemplating the hunger and fullness problem, I realized that some foods actually helped me recognize my own hunger and feelings of fullness. I began to identify them, calling them easy-to-manage foods, or easy foods for short. Easy-to-manage foods are attractive only when I am truly hungry. They are also easy to stop eating. When you look in the refrigerator and see an easy food, you might say to yourself, "That would be nice, but maybe later." I would skip these foods in favor of the foods I was highly attracted to.

The taste sensation provided by an easy-to-manage food is mildly stimulating rather than exciting. These foods keep the taste buds satisfied but calm. Easy foods can adequately satisfy the natural longings we have about food, but they don't compel us to overeat. Longings for sweet, salt, fat, crunchiness, and creaminess are acceptably met within the confines of easy-to-manage foods.

I suspect that, for normal eaters, most foods are easy-to-manage. For overeaters, far fewer foods fall into this category. The following are the easy-to-manage foods according to my own reactions. I hope that I'm average in my reactions, so that many overeaters can find this list very useful.

Easy-to-manage foods include:

Fruits:

Fresh or frozen fruit, canned fruit, applesauce, reconstituted dried fruit

Easy Dairy 4:

Milk, yogurt, cottage cheese, sour cream, and their non-dairy equivalents

Vegetables/Oil:

Steamed or sautéed vegetables, salad with dressing, vegetables with dip

Whole Starches:

Potatoes, beans, grains, rice, cooked cereal

Explanation of the preceding list:

Fruits—Any fresh, canned, or frozen fruit is an easy-to-manage food. Added sugar is fine, even the canned fruit in heavy syrup. Fruit, especially with added sugar, can satisfy that natural longing for sweet. Applesauce and other fruit sauces are easy-to-manage. Reconstituted dried fruit is also included. I'll explain my thoughts about dried fruit a little later.

Easy Dairy 4—Milk, yogurt, cottage cheese, and sour cream are the four easy-to-manage dairy foods. They may even be high in fat, such as sour cream. Easy dairy foods can satisfy the taste desire for creaminess, but they aren't overly attractive. They are very useful because they combine well with other easy foods. For example, yogurt and fruit go well together. Yogurt, juice, and fruit can be blended to make a smoothie. A dollop of cottage cheese in the middle of a dish of applesauce makes a mildly sweet/mildly salty treat. A sour-cream-based ranch dip is a nice accompaniment for raw veggies. Cooked cereals, such as oatmeal, are served with milk. A baked potato or a dish of lentils is deliciously topped by sour cream. Vegans or lactose intolerant individuals can take advantage of the soy and other non-dairy products that correspond to these foods.

Vegetables—Vegetables are also easy-to-manage foods. Salad vegetables provide crunchy chewing. Some of us have a great desire to chew, gnaw, and crunch. We often overeat because of this oral need. Notice that I separated potatoes from the vegetables and placed them in the whole starch category. They fill the same place in a meal as cooked grains and beans.

Vegetables also serve an important function in this list of easy foods. They can be vehicles for the oil and salt that we naturally crave. Vegetables may be sautéed in oil or sprinkled with oil dressing. Oil or fat helps greatly in hunger satisfaction and prevents that gnawing hunger we experience when our diet is too low in fat. I link vegetables with oil because oil can cause difficulty with the whole starch category that is next.

Whole Starches—Whole starches include potatoes, grains such as rice or cooked cereal, and dried beans. Typical offerings in this category are: baked or boiled potatoes, rice, baked beans, lentils, and oatmeal. The whole starches give that stick-to-the-ribs feeling and provide warmth to the body.

Whole starches are starchy foods that are usually steamed or boiled. The baked starches, such as bread, are placed in a different category. Do not confuse my use of the term "whole starch," with the term "whole grain."

When whole starches are prepared with generous amounts of oil or fat, the food becomes too attractive or overly stimulating to the taste buds. Under these conditions, the whole starch becomes a difficult-to-manage food. French fries and potato salad are prime examples of this. The commercial salty snack food items capitalize on this attraction to combined oil, salt, and starch.

It's tricky to categorize food. For example, I consider oil to be an easy-to-manage food as long as it is linked to vegetables. But what about mayonnaise and margarine? Both derive from vegetable oil. So, are they easy foods also? If you read on into the next section, you'll see how I tried to solve this predicament and others.

The easy-to-manage foods that I've listed could comprise a reasonably healthful diet. I doubt if anyone would overeat if their diet were made up of these choices. Easy foods just don't beckon unless you're truly hungry, and they get tiresome after hunger is satisfied. That type of feeling about food is important for overeaters to experience and appreciate. Yet, easy foods do satisfy the basic longings we have about food.

Easy-to-manage foods help us to know when we are hungry. You might say they are a litmus test for true hunger. If you don't want to eat an easy food, you really don't need to eat. Beware that you might *feel* hungry but still not want to eat an easy food. You might think the food is too boring, or you may be mildly repulsed at the thought of eating it. In either case, the hunger you're feeling is probably what I call first-stage hunger. I've come to understand that those initial feelings of hunger are not lasting. When the stomach empties out, we experience a hunger that soon passes. Then we can enjoy a delightful lightness. When real hunger returns, easy foods will once again start to look good to eat.

Easy foods also help us to know when to stop eating. It is hard to eat beyond fullness with easy-to-manage foods. They taste good at first, but as soon as you start to fill up, easy foods lose their attraction. This is a normal reaction. Don't give up on these foods because you experience this type of reaction. Remember, we're trying to develop normal reactions to food.

Difficult-to-manage foods

After a list of easy-to-manage foods was established, the remaining foods were labeled as difficult-to-manage. This is a large and varied group. Difficult-to-manage foods are the foods that are highly attractive even when we're not hungry. They are also hard to stop eating once we get started. Difficult foods need to be monitored in some way because they don't have the self-limiting quality of the easy-to-manage foods.

Difficult food easily trumps our genuine feelings of hunger and fullness. If we see a difficult food and it's available to eat, we're drawn to have at least a taste. Then the taste sensations lure us to keep eating. The taste of a difficult food is experienced as overly stimulating rather than mildly stimulating.

Difficult foods are not equal in their degree of difficulty. Some of them are the real problem foods that we might even say we feel addicted to. If given a choice, we always choose them. Some of the foods are far less difficult. Nevertheless, they are all gathered together under the heading of difficult-to-manage. I established four types of difficult foods.

Difficult-to-manage foods include:

Meat, Cheese, and Eggs:

Meats including fish, hard and soft cheese, eggs

Creamy Favorites:

Butter—and other spreads such as margarine, mayonnaise, cream cheese, cheese spread, peanut butter

Ice cream—and other desserts such as frozen yogurt, frozen custard, pudding

Whipped cream—and other toppings such as whipped topping, marshmallow

Flour Foods:

Cakes, pastries, cookies, bars

Donuts, coffee cake, croissants, muffins, scones, nut breads

French toast, biscuits, waffles, pancakes, ready-to-eat cereal

Pasta, noodles, dumplings, batter-dipped foods

Breads, bagels, rolls, pita, tortillas, crisp bread

Snack Foods:

Chips, pretzels, crackers, popcorn, puffed snacks

Candy: chocolate, caramel, butterscotch, fruit-flavored, licorice

Snack meats and cheeses, peanuts, nuts

Trail mix, granola bars, soy nuts, sunflower seeds, dried fruit

Explanation of the preceding list:

Meat, Cheese, Eggs—The first grouping of difficult foods consists of animal products that comprise the typical protein entrée. Meat stands for red meat, poultry, and fish. Cheese includes all types of hard and soft cheese, both high fat and low fat. A hard-boiled egg may not seem very difficult, but a fried egg can be very compelling.

Creamy Favorites—In this category I list a variety of foods that are similar in some way to butter, ice cream, and cream. Here is where I solved the margarine and mayonnaise problem. They, along with cream cheese and peanut butter, are listed as spreads which can take the place of butter. This is an irregular grouping of these foods. It is based on the way these foods are typically used in the diet. They all have a creamy texture and are highly attractive.

Soft serve, custard, sherbet, and frozen yogurt attempt to imitate high-fat ice cream. I decided to keep them together since I find all of them tempting regardless of fat content. Any of these can lure me away from a juice beverage like lemonade when I'm sitting at the drive-in window for an afternoon treat. Ice cream and its imitators get in the way of my choosing a beverage, which is the habit I want to form. Although not frozen, pudding is placed here as well. Sweetened milk—like the chocolate or strawberry milk that I said was too compelling to allow on my free choice beverage list—could be placed in this category. It's similar to melted ice cream.

Whipped cream is usually sweetened and is a difficult-to-manage food. Whipped toppings imitate the cream original and are just as difficult. I include marshmallow topping and marshmallows in this group as well. I know that overeaters sometimes like to keep a bag of marshmallows as a guilt-free sweet treat. However, this will keep your taste buds clamoring for more excitement, leading to further indulgence.

Flour Foods—The third type of difficult food is what I call the flour foods. They all include a highly processed grain, usually wheat flour. I listed the most difficult ones first, followed by less difficult examples.

It may seem unfair to cast a dry, wholegrain cracker into the same category as a frosted cupcake. But as soon as you cover a piece of crisp bread with a thin spread of butter, it becomes quite attractive. As a rule, the whole grain flour foods are easier-to-manage than the white flour foods. Certainly, bakery treats such as cookies, pastries, donuts, and cakes pose the greatest threat to overeaters.

The wide range of flour foods creates confusion, and with confusion comes temptation. One morning I would have a whole grain muffin for breakfast. The next morning someone in the family would make pancakes, and I'd think, "Why not have pancakes with a little butter and syrup? Is it so much different than a high fat bran muffin?" The morning after that, I am confronted by donuts, and I easily reason that a donut can't be any worse than the white flour pancakes I ate yesterday. Soon I'm facing a daily conflict with flour foods that wear me down and make me susceptible to temptation. Therefore, I decided to place all flour foods in the difficult-to-manage category.

As you can see, I list ready-to-eat cereal as a difficult flour food. The grain in these cereals is highly processed, like flour. Even the whole grain types are more attractive than cooked cereal. An overeater can easily consume two bowls of ready-to-eat cereal, but we wouldn't even think of eating two bowls of oatmeal at one sitting. The fun varieties of sugar-coated, ready-to-eat cereals are even more tempting and difficult-to-manage.

Certain types of bread can provide a chewy-ness that is rarely found in any of the easy-to-manage foods. Therefore, when I have bread I try to select chewy or crusty bread. Basic breads have been an important part of a simple diet throughout history. Bread was the original convenience food of great versatility. It could be baked and stored without refrigeration for future use. The people of many cultures rely upon some kind of bread for daily sustenance, and it still holds an honored place in the modern diet. The overeater, however, needs to be cautious when consuming bread.

Snack Foods—These foods greatly stimulate the taste buds. Rather than satisfying the normal taste urge, they create unnatural taste cravings. It's very hard to stop eating them once you start. Even if you think they really hit the spot and you feel satisfied, you'll return for another and another with increasing frequency. Before you know it, you'll be standing by the counter in a munching trance. They are extremely attractive, often using chemical enhancements and artificial flavors.

Snack foods are the real culprits of modern-day obesity. I believe the proliferation of salty snack food is probably the single greatest cause of childhood obesity. Candy and bakery treats have been available for centuries, but salty snack foods have only been widely available and popular in the past fifty years. These are the junk foods that dance off the shelves and into our grocery carts. They are the gas station foods, so easy to purchase and consume as we travel. They are ever expanding in variety and availability.

Salty snack foods include chips, popcorn, pretzels, salted nuts, snack meats, and snack cheeses. Salted crackers need to be included here as well. No matter how low fat or natural the snack item is touted to be, if it's convenient and salty, I need to avoid it.

Candy is just as prevalent as salty snack food. Chocolate candy is especially tempting for many people. Even fruit-flavored hard candy or other fat-free candy is a problem. Popping a jellybean here and there certainly isn't going to make anyone gain weight, but it reinforces the nibbling habit that leads to foods that are serious threats to health and cause excess fat. If you want some sugar, always have a sweet juice beverage, not a piece of candy. Like many overeaters, I've always had a weakness for chocolate. When I cheated on a diet, it inevitably included indulging in chocolate. I'd forgo lots of other delicious flavors if chocolate was available. I knew I needed to retrain my taste buds away from the chocolate obsession. Now, the less I eat chocolate, the less I enjoy the taste. With less exposure, the memory of the taste of chocolate actually fades. I have more freedom of choice if I avoid chocolate.

Healthful snack foods, I hate to say, are also difficult-to-manage. These presumably healthful alternatives often contain chocolate chips and other candies. Granola bars and trail mix, containing nuts, seeds and dried fruit, are too attractive to manage with ease. We try to do the right thing by choosing a granola bar rather than a candy bar. But it only ends up reminding us of the luscious chocolate bar that we really want. Trail mix encourages that mindless, hand-to-mouth munching that is very hard to stop once you start. Even dried fruit all by itself can be eaten in that trancelike way. Dried fruit gives that burst of concentrated flavor that is similar to candy. Nuts, seeds, and dried fruit are natural and nutritious, but they must be eaten cautiously.

Summary of beverages and foods

The following chart lists the types of beverages and foods I've been discussing. The three asterisks that appear in the chart are explained at the bottom. These asterisks refer to the three exceptions that were previously explained in more detail.

Summary of Beverages and Foods
Four Habits for Normal Eating

Beverages

Sweet: Apple juice and blends, grape juice, apricot nectar, hot cider

Tart: Orange juice, grapefruit juice, lemonade, cranberry cocktail

Salty: Tomato juice, vegetable juice

Protein: Milk*, soy milk, yogurt beverage

Water: Ice water, herbal tea, sparkling water*, (coffee, tea)

Easy-to-manage foods

Fruits:

Fresh or frozen fruit, canned fruit, applesauce, reconstituted dried fruit

Easy Dairy 4:

Milk, yogurt, cottage cheese, sour cream, and their non-dairy equivalents

Vegetables/Oil:

Steamed or sautéed vegetables, salad with dressing, vegetables with dip

Whole Starches:

Potatoes*, beans, grains, rice, cooked cereal

Difficult-to-manage foods

Meat, Cheese, and Eggs:

Meats including fish, hard and soft cheese, eggs

Creamy Favorites:

Butter—and other spreads such as margarine, mayonnaise, cream cheese, cheese spread, peanut butter

Ice cream—and other desserts such as frozen yogurt, frozen custard, pudding

Whipped cream—and other toppings such as whipped topping, marshmallow

Flour Foods:

Cakes, pastries, cookies, bars

Donuts, coffee cake, croissants, muffins, scones, nut breads

French toast, biscuits, waffles, pancakes, ready-to-eat cereal

Pasta, noodles, dumplings, batter-dipped foods

Breads, bagels, rolls, pita, tortillas, crisp bread

Snack Foods:

Chips, pretzels, crackers, popcorn, puffed snacks

Candy: chocolate, caramel, butterscotch, fruit-flavored, licorice

Snack meats and cheeses, peanuts, nuts

Trail mix, granola bars, soy nuts, sunflower seeds, dried fruit

*Exceptions: Sweetened milk, soft drinks, and high fat preparations of potatoes or other whole starches are difficult-to-manage choices.

Two decisions

After identifying all the foods I encountered as either easy-to-manage or difficult-to-manage, I began putting this knowledge to work on a daily basis. It felt good to be able to name any food that came my way as either easy or difficult. I felt more in control of my life. We're more vulnerable to something when we can't name it and put it in its proper place. Finally, I had some useful street smarts about food. I could quickly recognize which foods kept me safe and which foods led me into conflict.

When I chose what to eat, I did not restrict myself to easy foods because I still wanted to make room for the more stimulating but difficult foods. I considered abstaining from difficult foods, but I preferred to be able to move about freely in many eating situations. I did not want to make or request special accommodations to satisfy the demands of a restrictive eating plan. Therefore, I decided to simply rely upon easy-to-manage foods and reduce consumption of difficult-to-manage foods.

Easy foods are like the flat, steady rocks you encounter as you carefully cross the stream. Difficult foods are like the other rocks that are jagged and slippery. You need to use them once in a while, but seek out the reliable rocks. For ease of recall, here is an abbreviated listing of the four types of foods within each category:

Easy-to-manage foods	Difficult-to-manage foods
Fruits	Meat, Cheese, Eggs
Easy Dairy 4	Creamy Favorites
Vegetables/Oil	Flour Foods
Whole Starches	Snack Foods

I ate and drank throughout the day keeping in mind the two decisions I had made: 1) Rely on water and juice beverages between meals and 2) Rely on easy-to-manage foods for meals and reduce consumption of difficult-to-manage foods. These two decisions gave me a feeling of freedom and normality that I had long sought. I began to feel comfortable in the world of food. It was a relief not to have to monitor so closely how much I ate because my own body seemed much more responsive to hunger and fullness. My food cravings were also diminishing. I chose food that helped me feel like a normal eater rather than choosing food from a calorie, carbohydrate, or fat gram chart.

As I focused on easy foods, the difficult foods began to fade into the background. Everything tasted good, but nothing compelled me to take more than I needed. However, I admit I was somewhat disconcerted by the lack of taste excitement.

Nibbling keeps food cravings alive

Overeaters crave taste excitement. Some people crave salt while others have a sweet tooth. Many of us have both. We seesaw from one to the other. Although I was relying on juice beverages between meals to redirect taste desires, food cravings do not go down without a fight. I had to contend with a nibbling and tasting habit that kept food cravings alive.

Some overeaters taste and nibble on food all day. People who love to nibble have a hard time seeing any attractive food without reaching out for a taste. We constantly get up and look in the cupboard or refrigerator for a bite of food. The desire to eat invades every waking hour. We habitually seek small bursts of intense flavor.

Nibbling before and after a meal becomes more enjoyable than sitting down for the meal itself. By contrast, if a certain time is set aside to enjoy a tempting food, such as during suppertime, the tastes are enjoyed with greater perspective. It's far safer to indulge some snack food within the context of a meal than to have the food as an isolated snack.

In the days when taste cravings were a big problem for me, I remember trying to find some way to deal with that desire for intense flavor. First, I tried to suppress the desire by swearing off problem foods. That worked if I didn't count all the cheating I did. Then I tried designating one small salty or chocolate treat to eat whenever I wanted a tiny taste. I reasoned that I should try to satisfy the desire with something I really wanted. I figured if I had just a taste, the craving would go away. But nothing satisfied for long. That taste led only to more craving. Even the less attractive substitutions kept my taste buds persistently reawakening for another fix of intense flavor.

Food manufacturers know the weight-conscious nibbler very well. Makers of popular candy bars are now offering bags of bite-size pieces of their products. The dieter is drawn to the pleasure of taking a small taste of the flavor they crave. It seems sensible because the calorie count of that small piece won't wreck a diet, and it temporarily satisfies the clamoring taste urge. That bite, however, keeps your cravings alive and kicking. Soon, you'll be eating half the bag at a sitting. Those bites of candy will eventually undo whatever discipline you have for dieting.

I finally gave up trying to suppress or satisfy those pesky taste cravings. The harder I fought to find a solution to the problem, the stronger the problem seemed to become. It grew in proportion to the amount of effort I put into defeating it. I really needed to forsake the conflict and walk away. I know this is so much easier said than done. For many of us, this is the heart of the conflict. Time stands still as we stare into the snack cupboard and fight the urge to take "just a taste."

Food cravings can be habitual physical responses, especially at certain times of the day. If you can successfully interrupt the habit a few times, it will lose power. The sum total of the positive efforts you make to feel like a normal eater will give you the ability to succeed. Even better, these efforts will help you to completely avoid food cravings. Remember: Keep redirecting taste desires with juice and fully satisfying thirst with water. This is a helpful strategy for salt cravings as well as sugar cravings. Both salt and sugar cravings are habitual and driven by thirst.

If you want a snack rather than a beverage, try nature's original snack food—fruit. It won't excite your taste buds, but it will taste very good. Fruit won't immediately defeat your intense food cravings, but this is a positive action to take when you're harassed by the desire to nibble. The more you turn to fruit snacks, the more your body will respond favorably to fruit. I remember being surprised the first time I went through a snack buffet line and discovered I was drawn to the fruit. The salty cheeses and buttery snack crackers didn't tempt me as much. It's wonderful when the body responds and begins to support the choices you've consciously made. The body will want what it is used to having. What a relief not to have to fight and deny what you want, because you actually desire the better choice!

Many overeaters have eaten very little fruit because it does not provide the taste excitement they crave. You may even believe you don't like fruit. This dislike of fruit might be a food prejudice that developed in childhood. Some fruit may not agree with you, especially at certain times of the day, yet other fruits may suit you. If a piece of fresh fruit makes your teeth feel funny, have canned fruit instead. It's not necessary to eat a large serving of fruit. If you can't eat a whole pear, eat just a few pieces. If you try to eat the whole pear, you could be thoroughly sick of it before you're done. Train yourself with small amounts.

Fruit also comes in handy for the overeaters among us who are not nibblers and tasters. Some overeaters have very little trouble with between-meal snacking, but once they start eating during a meal, they have a hard time stopping. These hearty eaters have a much easier time ending their meal if they have an attractive dessert to look forward to. A nice fruit-filled dessert is a real benefit to them. Apple crisp, peach cobbler, and cherry pie are examples of fruit-filled desserts. These should not be heavily indulged or eaten between meals, because they are difficult-to-manage. But, a moderate portion provides a celebratory conclusion to a meal and is very helpful to the hearty eater.

The snack cupboard

For those of us sharing our home with others, it's hard to forsake snack food when people all around us are eating freely of it. If you are always encountering snack food, you'll be thrown right back into conflicts with food.

I would have loved to keep all snack foods out of the house. But since I had a family, I had to find ways to adapt to the presence of snack foods. Most importantly, I keep them off the counter tops and relegated to one cupboard. I try not to open that cupboard except with the intent of clearing out and throwing away old snacks. I avoid looking at them or bumping into them. If they're out of sight, they're out of mind. It's not easy, but it is possible to peacefully coexist with troublesome foods.

Food invasions are a regular part of family life. One child brings home a case of candy that they are required to sell for a school fundraiser. Another child needs to bring tortilla chips to a gathering, and half a bag comes home along with other leftover treats. The neighbor drops off a plate of cookies. Your mother brings leftover chocolate cake from her women's club. Food invasions get wildly out of control during the holidays. A difficult food invasion can completely undermine your self-control.

Put those invading foods in the snack cupboard for a short period of time; then, do not hesitate to throw them out. Frugality serves no good purpose with problem foods. The longer they hang around, the more you start to think the only way to get rid of them is to eat. If the food hasn't been eaten within the span of one week, normal eaters in the family will never get around to it. Eventually, the overeaters will devour it in a weak moment or to finally rid themselves of the temptation. It's far better to throw out the invading food than to eat it. You could give it away, but to whom? Definitely not to a fellow overeater! Normal eaters won't accept it, because they know it'll just sit on their counter. The only reasonable option is to bring the food to a group gathering or to a large family of skinny children.

The fruit-filled desserts that I spoke of earlier are not kept in the snack cupboard. I don't like to mix these acceptable desserts with the troublesome snack foods. They'll stay fresher tasting in the refrigerator, and freshness, by the way, is important. Over-eaters will eat something for fear it won't taste fresh tomorrow. Always remember, these fruit-filled desserts should be eaten as a dessert, not as a between-meal snack.

When you intentionally buy some snack food for your family, it's best to keep the snack food fairly monotonous. For your children, keep one standard cookie that they like and they feel good about offering to their friends. Don't purchase the latest cookie to hit the market. You will be interested in trying it, and they'll probably eat more than they normally would. If you keep salty snack food, keep one type of chip or cracker that everyone likes. The secret to managing snacks is not to vary the stock. Find out what your family members really want in the snack cupboard. Then stick to it. Do not vary it. The variety of foods we face today is a major problem for the overeater.

The need to limit choice

Increased choice and availability of food in modern life make us even more vulnerable to overeating. If we lived one hundred years ago, chances are most of us would not be overeating nearly as much as we are today. There just wasn't the expansive choice and certainly not the convenience of many foods. If you wanted some ice cream, you had to crank for it instead of simply reaching into the grocery store freezer for one of many varieties of ice cream. Nowadays, food is everywhere, just waiting for us to plunk down our money and carry it away to eat.

New food products hit the market every week to jazz up our lives, keep us interested, and keep us consuming. Endless variety fosters confusion and weakness in the overeater. We easily become distracted from our self-control decisions when faced with too many choices. We all know what it is like to feel full, then suddenly able to eat again, when a new and interesting food is offered. Even normal eaters consume more when faced with a buffet table laden with food.

The need to limit choice gave rise to my third decision. I began to rely upon a simple meal guide to cope with ever-increasing food variety. I wanted my meal guide to give helpful structure to my meal decisions, just as the beverage path gave structure to my between-meal decisions.

I will present my daily meal guide later and give a detailed explanation on how to apply it in different situations. It is necessary to examine it closely because many carefully constructed eating plans flounder in the rush of life. Many plans that look good on paper suddenly become unworkable when you're out in the everyday world. Some people will be able to use my guide, but others will need to construct their own.

A meal guide will direct your choices, but it should be flexible enough to fit into most eating situations. It should allow you to emphasize the easy-to-manage foods without taking you out of the mainstream of life. It should not make you stand out from the crowd. You may have seen someone at a banquet being served, by special request, a meal that is different from everyone else's food. Some people might not mind the attention they receive by eating something different from others in the group, but that kind of attention is excruciating to many of us. Your meal guide should be like a comfortable suit of clothes, not a straightjacket. It should be a valuable aid rather than an annoying restriction.

The ideal meal guide fits easily into your lifestyle and culture. It should help you cut through the confusing and clamoring food choices you face. It reduces the number of food decisions you have to make each day, thus allowing you to turn your attention to other matters and pleasurable pursuits.

Spiritual disciplines and food

There are spiritual advantages to keeping food choice limited. Most of the world's people eat simple, humble fare. Food variety is both a blessing and a curse on the wealthy peoples of the world. The eating of basic foods can create a feeling of oneness with the majority of the people inhabiting our planet. Countless numbers of our brothers and sisters under God have eaten the same humble food day after day. Is it so difficult for us to do likewise? Simplicity of food is a time-honored part of the spiritual life.

The practice of abstaining from certain foods is often used as spiritual discipline. In modern times, people also abstain for ethical or health reasons. For example, one might abstain from meat out of moral convictions. Others abstain from foods they feel are not healthful, such as sugar, wheat, or milk. Some people respond well to the rigors of abstaining. Abstaining has a rather noble feel to it. The act of abstaining can also provide a sense of solidarity with people who are dealing with temptations like alcoholism and smoking where abstinence is the necessity.

I considered abstaining from certain of the most difficult-to-manage foods. But I quickly found that, for me, abstaining gives the identified food more power. I found it very hard to surrender to the finality of abstinence with regard to any food. Food is so much more benign than other substances of abuse; it doesn't seem to warrant total abstinence. I didn't like making any food a "forbidden fruit" because it only seemed to increase the conflict of temptation. Thus, I chose to reduce consumption of difficult food rather than abstain. I looked past the difficult food whenever possible. I preferred to focus on the simple, easy-to-manage foods while allowing difficult food simply to fade into the background.

Fasting, the act of abstaining from all food for a day or so, is another ancient spiritual discipline. Fasting can be an instructive experience. It makes you aware of how dependent you are, not only on food, but also on the daily rituals of food. I often toyed with the idea of fasting each day from 7:00 PM to 7:00 AM, ending with a true *break-fast*. There are some important benefits to this half-day fast, including being able to sleep better. But again, I found that it was better for me to take a less rigorous approach. Now I just tell myself that it's good to have some consumption-free times and let it go at that. I try to remember to rely solely on water and breath at various times during the day.

Just breathe

It is important for overeaters to remember that food isn't the primary life-sustaining substance. Before we need food, we need water. Before we need water, we need air. I've said that the overeater misinterprets thirst and turns to food. Similarly, our need to breathe well can be misdirected to food.

Overeaters must learn to feel at home with just breathing. Somewhere along the line, we started thinking we must have something else besides air to consume most of the time. This may have begun because we got used to constantly sipping a diet soda or even the healthful alternative of bottled water. It's possible we started to sprinkle our day with those bursts of flavor from tasting and nibbling between meals. Perhaps we tried the diet strategy of eating many small meals, and those meals disintegrated into continuous snacking. No matter how this pattern began, we need to develop a sense of satisfaction from the consumption of air in relaxed breathing.

Relaxed breathing stimulates attention, improves concentration, and promotes clarity of thought. We get a feeling of unification or centeredness when we breathe well. This goes a long way toward helping the overeater feel a sense of dignity and calm. We achieve relaxed alertness without utilizing food.

Breathing well is very important for keeping an internal balance of calmness and alertness. Breath, however, is ignored when we eat to calm down and relax the nerves. We also eat to keep ourselves alert, or even awake. Often we turn to crunchy and chewy food for this purpose. Unfortunately, the crunchy snack foods rather than crunchy vegetables or fruit are the most attractive and readily available for this purpose. If you find yourself rummaging through the snack cupboard, you may need to stop and take a deep breath.

Good breathing also helps moderate the physical effects of emotional stress. Emotional eating plays a large role in the overeating tendencies of many people. Overeaters often eat more when stressed, while normal eaters may eat less under those same conditions. The spiritual practices described in this book will help far more than physical techniques for alleviating emotional distress and even preventing it. However, physical interventions can help. I mentioned earlier that I sip cold water to ease the internal heat of emotional stress. It is well known that exercise reduces the strain of emotional pressure. Similarly, deep breathing mitigates the physical stress brought on by difficult emotions.

Beware of nervous habits such as nail biting, hair twisting, leg jiggling, or finger tapping, to name just a few. While you're doing those things, you're probably not breathing well. We develop nervous habits for the same reason that we eat to obtain the alert/calm state. Rather than being effective, they contribute to a feeling of disintegration instead of the unified, balanced feeling that we seek.

A state of relaxed alertness is the ideal physical state. For anyone familiar with the practice of meditation, that perfect balance of calmness and alertness characterizes the experience. The feeling called "flow," in work or play, also produces this balance. Scientific research has investigated whether foods promote mood changes, particularly in the area of calmness and alertness. If nerves are on edge, the consumption of carbohydrates may help to calm us. If we feel lethargic, a protein food may be just the stimulation we need. Therefore, reaching for food isn't completely off target. The trouble is, we usually overdo it, thereby canceling the effectiveness of the food being consumed for that purpose.

Take a little time to work on your breathing. Relearn how to breathe fully, completely, and comfortably. Periodically, I will lie down and relax the muscles in my face, neck, and chest until my breathing normalizes. There are books on breathing that can help you locate your particular breathing problem. For me, I found that I needed to consciously expand the bottom of my lungs to let air reach into the entire lung space. Then I fully exhale and relax down into the pause between breaths.

Try doing some stretching exercises, and focus on your breathing while you do them. Just a few minutes of practice each day will help. Any type of exercise helps us to breathe better, inhaling and exhaling for full oxygenation of our cells. An exercise such as yoga can refresh the mind as well as ease stress. Physical exertion rids the body of nervous tension. Movement warms the body and brings on pleasurable feelings of youthfulness and well-being. Moderate exercise can energize as well as relax.

Good breathing helped me in ways I did not expect. I felt less tired and sore in the evening. It helped some chronic middle-back problems that would show up in late afternoon. It also improved my attention and focus for reading. It definitely helped me to sleep better. A few minutes of good breathing can be an excellent way to prepare the body for sleep.

Make sure you're getting enough sleep. With more people getting less sleep due to the fast pace of modern life, overeating for this reason could be widespread. The act of eating counteracts feelings of fatigue, and you may be using it to stay awake. You just might be eating when you should be sleeping. A well-rested body is of great help in naturally achieving the calmness and alertness that are integral to a productive and healthy life.

Breath is where the spiritual, mental, and physical disciplines meet. Breath is essential to the body. Good breathing enhances mind mastery. We refer to the Spirit as the breath of life. When you practice good breathing, take advantage of this connection. Try linking your breath with a prayerful phrase that is meaningful to your spiritual life. Remember that the body is the temple of God, and the mind is the sanctuary of the divine presence.

When you sit down for a meal, take a relaxed breath before you eat. Survey your food with appreciation and feel a sense of abundance. Admire the display of food and take time to smell the aromas. Remember those who labored to provide this sustenance. And give thanks to God, who is the source of all life and energy.

Breath and soft drinks

I mentioned earlier that I would address the problem of soft drinks again. Only when I understood the importance of relying on breath did I stop depending upon my favorite soft drink. I noticed that I actually breathed better during those first sips of soda. The carbonated beverage reminded me or caused me to relax and breathe. That may be part of the reason I came to depend upon soft drinks. I needed to breathe, but I misinterpreted that need as longing for soft drinks.

I also realized that I used cola as a crutch to help me through those times of nonconsumption when I should have been just breathing. Overeaters feel that they always need to be consuming something. This is especially true if you've dieted a lot. We cling to that sugar-free soda in our anxiety about food and fear of feeling hungry.

Gradually, I stopped depending on soft drinks. For a long time, I would turn to my favorite cola only for emergency stress reduction. I reasoned that it was far better for me to reach for a soda than to start snacking in response to stress. And that was true. It was a step forward for me to do that. But eventually, my favorite cola lost its appeal. Since I didn't drink it on a daily basis, it began to taste strange to me. After this transition, I began to rely upon cold water and, more importantly, good breathing to reduce the physical effects of stress.

Four habits for normal eating

Based on what I learned about variety of food and breath, I added two more decisions to the two I had already made. I decided to rely on a simple menu guide to prevent the confusion and weakness brought on by variety. Lastly, I decided to rely on breath for relaxed alertness as well as physical and emotional stress reduction. This brought me to a total of four decisions, as follows:

1. Rely on water and juice beverages between meals to redirect taste desires and diminish food cravings that thirst intensifies.

2. Rely on easy-to-manage foods for meals and reduce consumption of difficult-to-manage foods to improve hunger/fullness recognition and naturally reduce food consumption.

3. Rely on a simple meal guide to cope with the increased choice and availability of food in modern life.

4. Rely on breath to achieve relaxed alertness and decrease stress-induced eating.

With these four decisions, I felt a sense of stability I hadn't had before. I could depend on these decisions when times were tough. They could become solid, life-affirming habits. Many eating plans can only be followed when we're mentally sharp and in a good mood. When hard times come, the plan becomes an extra burden that adds to the stress we are already feeling from other sources.

On the basis of these four decisions, I constructed the *Four Habits for Normal Eating*. In this plan, strong taste desires, which are intensified by unrecognized thirst, are reduced and redirected. Hunger and fullness sensitivity is improved by the mild taste stimulation of the easy-to-manage foods. Everyday food selections become less confusing, and good breathing assists in stress reduction. Through these techniques, we begin to feel more like normal eaters. We start to experience genuine self-control amid the temptation of food.

This plan is corrective because underlying physical causes of overeating are addressed. Too often, we ignore these causes in the rush to lose weight. Each habit redirects behavior into a positive action that alleviates the physical cause. The following chart summarizes the four habits and provides a brief definition of easy-to-manage foods as well as difficult-to-manage foods.

Four Habits for Normal Eating

1. **Rely on water and juice beverages between meals**—to redirect taste desires and diminish food cravings that thirst intensifies.

2. **Rely on easy-to-manage foods for meals and reduce consumption of difficult-to-manage foods**—to improve hunger/fullness recognition and naturally reduce food consumption.

3. **Rely on a simple meal guide**—to cope with the increased choice and availability of food in modern life.

4. **Rely on breath**—to achieve relaxed alertness and decrease stress-induced eating.

Easy-to-manage foods are attractive when you're truly hungry. **Difficult-to-manage foods** are highly attractive even when you're not hungry.

Easy-to-manage foods	Difficult-to-manage foods
Fruits	Meat, Cheese, Eggs
Easy Dairy 4	Creamy Favorites
Vegetables/Oil	Flour Foods
Whole Starches	Snack Foods

A daily beverage and meal guide

The meal guide, in addition to the beverage path, provides daily structure for the four habits. It reminds me when and what to eat and drink as I make my way through the day. It keeps me focused on the foods and beverages that are helpful and satisfying choices at certain times of the day. I use this same plan each day. It helps me to remember what works well, but I know I can be flexible with it. This guide is specifically designed to suit me. If you should choose to use this guide, it can be altered to accommodate your own preferences, lifestyle, and special needs.

The middle column of the following chart, the beverage path, includes the sweet, tart, and salty beverages that are so important for training taste desires. Water should be drunk freely throughout the day. Water beverages, such as herbal tea, are scheduled in the path. If I want a snack in addition to beverages between meals, I rely on fruits or easy dairy.

The third column, the meal guide, lists my usual three meals. Fruit, easy dairy, and a whole starch like oatmeal provide a good start to a day of normal eating. Lunch and supper are dominated by vegetables and, whenever possible, the whole starches. You probably have questions about the veggie-filled sandwich and what I mean by the suppertime main dish. Please read on for a complete explanation of this meal guide and how I adapt it for various situations.

*

A Daily Beverage and Meal Guide Four Habits for Normal Eating		
Time of Day	**Beverage Path**	**Meal Guide**
Breakfast	Water* Coffee	Fruit, Milk, Oatmeal
Mid-morning	Fruit herb tea Sweet juice	
Lunch		Veggie-filled Sandwich
Mid-afternoon	Tea Tart juice	
Supper	Salty juice	Vegetables and Main Dish Fruit-filled Dessert
Evening	Milk Mint herb tea	

  * Fruits and Easy Dairy are recommended for snacks.
  * Drink water freely throughout the day.

The devil is in the details

Now, I would like to embark on a detailed explanation of how I actually put the beverage and meal guide to work from morning to night. I've made the explanation as complete as possible because, as the old saying goes, "the devil is in the details." I've found that a seemingly small ambiguity or problem within an eating plan can cause a big disruption. Just as a personal fitness trainer makes an exercise plan and then watches carefully to make corrections on how the client does the exercises, so must we be our own eating trainer, identifying small problems and making corrections for the success of the eating plan. The following explanation is fine-tuned to meet my needs, which I hope are fairly typical.

Early morning and breakfast

Like many people, I drink coffee in the morning. But first, I have at least six ounces of water so that I'm not drinking coffee to quench thirst. In addition, too much caffeine can cause me to start eating in order to calm my nerves.

My usual breakfast consists of milk, fruit, and cereal. Cooked cereal is the easy-to-manage choice. If you miss your favorite ready-to-eat cereal, perhaps eat it every other day. However, keep trying to get used to a less processed, hot cereal like oatmeal. As is often the case, we want what we are used to having. Cooked cereal, because of its water content, feels far more satisfying on much less. I use one-quarter cup rolled oats to make a bowl of oatmeal for myself. That much granola would look pitiful in the bowl.

I like canned peaches in heavy syrup as the breakfast fruit. It's always available and always good tasting. I mention heavy syrup because many overeaters might not choose fully sweetened canned fruit in order to avoid sugar calories. Early on, I decided I wasn't going to be overly concerned about sugar. The longing for sweet flavor is natural and basic to existence. For those who prefer less sweet, the light syrups are certainly available. Fresh fruit in season is a breakfast treat to be cherished. However, off-season, it may be disagreeably crunchy or not sweet enough. Wonderful fresh fruits are increasingly available in larger cities, but if you live in a small town or can't get to the store very often, your best bet may be canned fruit.

At some point, I started to skip the cooked cereal. That caused me to be hungry later in the morning, making me vulnerable to snacks. I finally realized I was skipping it because I didn't feel like making the oatmeal. I was in the habit of making oatmeal in a pan over the stove. As soon as I recognized the problem, I started microwaving it and have been happily eating oatmeal ever since. This is just one example of how a small, unidentified problem can sabotage an eating plan.

The best difficult foods to bring in are those that combine well with easy foods. For example, I occasionally have pancakes topped with sweetened strawberries and vanilla yogurt. Pancakes are an acceptable substitute for the oatmeal so long as there is a strong fruit presence.

Make sure to have some fat with breakfast. The fat I have for breakfast usually comes in the form of half and half that I use liberally in coffee and sometimes on oatmeal. Fat during a meal prevents that gnawing hunger feeling later. I usually buy two percent milk, but I enjoy whole milk if it is offered to me. I find I need an adequate combination of protein, starch, and fat in order to feel satisfied during any meal.

When I find myself rushing out of the house in the morning, with no time for breakfast, I grab a fruit-filled snack bar and buy a carton of milk. There is no use thinking this is never going to happen, so you might as well be prepared. I keep a box of these breakfast bars in the cupboard for that purpose. If they're individually wrapped, they'll stay fresh for those emergencies.

If I'm out for a sociable breakfast, cafes usually list oatmeal on the menu, and some may even offer pancakes with real fruit topping. In general, breakfast is the hardest meal to eat out. It can be depressing at first to look past the breakfast offerings of eggs, cheese, salty meat, fried potatoes, and various types of bakery treats. I told myself that if I really wanted to indulge those foods for old time's sake, I'd order them for supper rather than starting my day with them. Now that I'm more used to eating easy-to-manage foods, I rarely desire those types of breakfasts.

At a cafeteria or coffee bar, it's easy to find a dish of fresh fruit pieces as well as milk or yogurt. For starch, think bakery with fruit inside, preferably not shockingly high in fat. I might choose a blueberry scone or apricot biscotti. I usually look past the bagels because I save them for a lunch option.

If I'm in a fast-food restaurant, I look for yogurt with fresh fruit and granola sprinkles. They also might offer ready-to-eat cereal. I've certainly been known to give up and order milk and the basic breakfast sandwich. But this is risky, mainly because it gets me off the fruit-dairy-grain track and onto a salty food track in the morning. I prefer to start the day with a good dose of the taste training foods.

Some fast-food places offer smoothies for breakfast. Commercial smoothies are not always prepared with yogurt or whole fruit, and they may have far less protein than you expect for a meal. However, at least they keep your taste buds on track with fruit flavors.

I remind myself to sip a small amount of cold water after meals, including breakfast. This is done to settle and destimulate the digestive system after eating. I keep a bottle of water in the refrigerator for that purpose, or I prepare a glass of ice water. This technique is most effective if I'm mindful of the cold water as it travels down the esophagus into my stomach.

Mid-morning

I prefer a fruit herb tea like cranberry-apple in the morning. This time of day I don't like spicy or leafy-tasting teas. A fruit-dominated flavor fits in well with my morning food choices. If it is summertime and a hot beverage is not desired, I steep the tea in a half-filled, twelve-ounce mug, then add cold water and ice. If I think ahead, I can make sun tea.

Apricot nectar is my favorite sweet juice choice. Sometimes I'll drink it in a glass filled with ice to lighten the flavor and sweetness. If I get busy and forget to drink some, which is more often than not, I'll have a small glass as I'm fixing lunch. I want to keep training myself to seek fruit flavors and beverages between meals.

Lunch

Lunch was a problem for years. At noon, I'm low on energy and can't think straight. I would always plan to have a virtuous lunch of soup and salad. But so often, I would find myself nibbling my way through the noon hour rather than sitting down and eating a sensible lunch. I finally had to admit I felt deprived at the thought of only having soup and salad.

The standard, healthful lunch pattern in this culture includes soup, salad, and a sandwich. Since I was unhappy with just soup and salad, I figured I'd better find a sandwich that was fairly easy-to-manage. A veggie-filled sandwich like a submarine fits that description. If it is filled with lots of raw veggies and stacked with lesser amounts of cheese or meat, I consider it an acceptable easy-to-manage choice, almost like having a salad on a bun. The sub is satisfyingly chewy, and even the smaller, six-inch size looks like a substantial sandwich.

Before I developed this eating plan, I didn't like sub sandwiches. All those vegetables annoyed me because they reduced the taste stimulation of the salty meat and cheese that I craved. Now I know that, to eat normally, one does not expect food to hyperstimulate the taste buds.

At home, I don't keep all the sub sandwich ingredients on hand, so I have a variation. I usually have a small bagel with cream cheese and plenty of green leaf lettuce as the filling. For freshness, I buy frozen bagels, keep them in the freezer, then thaw one each day for lunch. Thin, sliced, red bell pepper or cucumber can also serve as a sandwich filler. Any type of chewy bread can substitute for the bagel. Carrot and celery sticks on the side, with a dab of sour-cream ranch dip, add nutrition and crunchy munching.

At lunchtime, I like to satisfy that need to crunch and chew by eating raw vegetables and chewy bread. I notice it if I don't have that crunching, chewing time each day. It has become an important measure for snacking prevention.

If I'm in a cafeteria, a beautiful salad bar makes a soup and salad lunch look tempting. At the salad bar, I avoid the pasta salads. Instead, I choose the garden vegetables topped with beans such as chickpeas. An oil dressing is best, but I think it's fine to choose any type of dressing you want. I usually choose a full-fat ranch dressing served on the side so I can dip my fork into it for each mouthful. As for soup, I look for one that features vegetables along with smaller amounts of difficult-to-manage ingredients like meat or noodles. It's unlikely that any soup will cause you to overeat because it is so high in liquid. Even cream soups are fine as long as they aren't so thick you could eat them with a fork. Potato soup and bean soup make good use of the whole starches. A soup and salad lunch, like this, actually became more appealing after I stopped requiring myself to have it.

The typical fast-food place, specializing in hamburgers and French fries, is the hardest place to find easy-to-manage food. Dieters stand confused, staring at the overhead menu, wishing they could just order a combo and be done with it. It used to be disappointing, and even mildly embarrassing, to order a soup and salad in such a place. The salad usually consisted of colorless lettuce with a worn-out tomato slice. The soup was salty and tasteless, dripping down the sides of a Styrofoam bowl. Ordering soup and salad in a fast-food restaurant made me feel like I was "on a diet." Thankfully, the major fast-food places are trying to offer more appealing salads, soups, and other healthful choices like baked potatoes.

Despite the better choices in fast-food places, I longed to be able to order a typical meal. So, what to do? I usually order a deluxe hamburger, consisting of a regular-size patty with lettuce and tomato. With a stretch of the imagination, I can see it as a veggie-filled sandwich. I order a noncarbonated sweet beverage like fruit punch to drink before consuming the meal. If I fill the cup to the brim with ice, I won't drink too much. To round out the order, I can purchase a side salad or soup. I appreciate it when a fast-food place offers a side salad or soup as a standard combo option. It's nice to be able to place a simple order and not have to search the overhead menu for separate items.

To end lunch, make sure to sip some ice water or take along a bottle of refrigerated water to sip in the car. It cools the digestive tract and provides a ritual with which to end the meal. Take a few good breaths, and if you can, relax a bit after lunch.

Mid-Afternoon

I look to tart flavors rather than sweet in the afternoon. Tart beverages include citrus drinks such as lemonade, grapefruit juice, and orange juice. When oranges and grapefruit are in season, I might have them in place of the juice. I also like to drink black tea in the mid-afternoon. The traditional black tea with lemon fits in nicely with the emphasis on tart flavors. In the summertime, I might have a glass of sweetened, lemon-flavored tea. Yogurt, even sweetened yogurt, tastes rather tart to me, so I prefer to have yogurt as an afternoon snack rather than at breakfast time.

I allow and actually encourage myself to eat fruit and easy dairy at any time of day, not just for breakfast. Fruit is the taste treat of the natural world, just right for snacking. Easy dairy supports these fruits and fruit flavors. I particularly like to keep applesauce and cottage cheese on hand. Cottage cheese is helpful when you want something mildly salty. By the way, I purchase the four percent cottage cheese because it tastes much better. A fresh apple is great when I want a crunchy fruit. Raw veggies fill that need for something crunchy also, but if I have veggies between meals, they won't be so attractive to me at lunch or supper, which is when I need to rely upon them.

Afternoon is a good time to have a fruit-flavored icy drink, a frozen whole fruit bar, or an occasional smoothie. As mentioned before, exercise some caution because the smoothie might be made from a frozen dairy confection like soft-serve or custard, thus making it more attractive. Wherever there are smoothies, there may also be ice cream. Many of us have bad diet memories of ordering a sugar-free cola when everyone else ordered a cone. Now, if I'm with a group of people, I usually order a cone along with everyone else. When choosing a flavor, I try to stay away from chocolate and flavors that include salty nuts or candy. Strawberry ice cream is the best choice because of the fruit flavor. It surprised me that ice cream lost much of its appeal when I took chocolate ice cream off the list of choices.

Supper

While fixing supper, I'll often have tomato juice or some other type of salty vegetable juice. It serves as an appetizer and starts to satisfy natural salt desires before eating the meal. As an alternative, I might drink a tart juice before supper, especially if the meal I'm preparing has a tomato sauce in it.

If I'm a guest at a dinner party or in a nice restaurant, I'll have an alcoholic beverage along with everyone else. However, I avoid the appetizers, even the healthful appetizers like vegetable dippers. If I start eating veggies before dinner, I'll be bored with them by the time the meal actually begins.

At suppertime, there is a large range of choice, which is nice but can be confusing to the overeater. There are two types of meals: the divided plate meal and the main dish meal.

The divided plate meal includes the dieter's typical meal consisting of a filet of grilled chicken or fish, along with a baked potato and steamed veggies. Following the usual advice, we can envision a picnic plate with three preformed sections. Place the vegetables in the large section. Then place the entrée in one of the smaller sections, and a whole starch in the other small section. This makes the divided plate meal conform to the idea of relying on easy-to-manage foods and reducing consumption of difficult-to-manage foods.

Since we don't always eat a divided plate meal, I need to discuss the varied options for main dishes. Examples of main dish meals can be listed in the following three groups:

1. Soup, stew, and main dish garden salad

2. Rice bowl, pasta bowl, noodle bowl, and casseroles

3. Pizza, tacos, and hot sandwiches

I prefer to prepare main dish meals that I can ladle or scoop into a bowl. The ideal bowl food consists primarily of vegetables and whole starches plus smaller amounts of difficult ingredients like meat or creamy sauces. The reason I prefer bowl food is that the mixture of foods reduces the stimulation of any difficult food in the dish. If you have a pleasant combination of vegetables, starch, and meat, the overall effect is much easier-to-manage than if the meat stood alone, as with the divided plate meal. The mixture is usually immersed in a broth or sauce to blend flavors. The broth or sauce also adds more liquid, which helps with fullness awareness.

The easiest-to-manage bowl foods are soups, stews, and salads. An example of a good soup choice would be a beef barley soup with plenty of vegetables. Chili with meat and plenty of beans serves as a good example of a thick soup or stew. A typical suppertime salad is a Caesar salad with grilled chicken. I mentioned earlier that I was unhappy about having soup and salad for lunch. That is not true for supper. I am quite happy to have a main dish soup or main dish salad for supper.

The second group of main dishes begins with the rice bowl. It is the easiest-to-manage of this group. The typical rice bowl consists of stir-fried vegetables and chicken over a bed of rice. Rice can also be topped by a cream sauce of vegetables and meat such as turkey. Mexican beans and rice may be placed here. Rice casseroles and rice salads are fine so long as they are not overloaded with difficult ingredients such as cheese or mayonnaise.

I need to be more cautious with the other bowl foods in the second group. Pasta bowls or noodle bowls consist primarily of a flour food that is difficult-to-manage. Bear in mind, a tomato sauce over pasta is easier-to-manage than a cheesy Alfredo sauce. I continue to prepare the standard spaghetti with meat sauce, but I like to place cooked spinach and cottage cheese next to it in the bowl. These easy-to-manage foods, eaten with the spaghetti, keep the stimulation moderate and complement the main dish. I also need to be cautious with pasta salads, which usually contain generous amounts of mayonnaise. To counter that in my own preparations, I keep the dressing minimal and substitute a reduced-fat sour cream for half the mayonnaise. I regularly serve a tuna pasta salad with lots of celery and peas.

Casseroles may consist of loose casseroles—that may be scooped into a bowl—or baked dishes like lasagna that are cut into squares and served on a plate. Square-cut baked dishes are usually held together with eggs and contain a substantial amount of cheese. In general, I consider loose casseroles to be easier-to-manage than the square-cut baked dishes. I look for casseroles that contain generous portions of easy-to-manage ingredients, such as beans, potatoes, and vegetables. One may argue that a meatless spinach lasagna is less difficult than a loose casserole containing meat. Such is the slippery nature of trying to categorize food. Despite these inconsistencies, I settled on the bowl food idea as something for me to aim for when choosing a main dish.

If you have a family, you're probably going to end up serving fun food like pizza, tacos, and hamburgers. Certainly, they are more difficult-to-manage than the bowl foods. They are even attractive enough to be eaten as snack foods. Anything you can do to add vegetables to these foods will make them a little easier-to-manage. A veggie pizza, a vegetarian sandwich, and a bean burrito with plenty of lettuce and tomato are your best options in this group.

I don't always have dessert. I think this is because I'm much more of a nibbler than a hearty eater. For hearty eaters, it's almost essential to include a fruit-filled dessert as a pleasant ending to a meal. This makes it easier for the hearty eater to stop eating. If I find myself in front of the dessert cart, I choose the fruit pie or the strawberry shortcake rather than the chocolate cream pie or the frosting topped cake. At least I'm reinforcing the natural and appropriate desire for fruit.

If you prefer a lighter dessert, substitute a dish of berries for the fruit-filled dessert. If only frozen berries are available, take some berries out to thaw during last-minute supper preparations. They'll be icy but soft when you're ready for dessert. Top them with some sprinkled sugar to bring out the flavor. Canned pears topped with vanilla yogurt and sprinkled with chopped walnuts make an easy, elegant dessert. If you have time, prepare a fruit salad with a lemon yogurt dressing for dessert.

Suppertime ends as I sip ice water to settle down. Drinking water after supper also helps to prevent snacking due to unrecognized thirst later on in the evening.

Evening

I used to end meals with a glass of milk, but now I have it as an evening beverage. Although I thoroughly enjoy milk, I still have to remind myself to drink it. When I do, it always has a good effect on me. It redirects that ice cream craving that comes around in the evening. It heads off other taste desires as well. If I go out at night, I usually save the milk to help me unwind when I get home.

After filling a glass with milk, I usually put water on to boil for tea. This milk- and-tea ritual has prevented many an evening snack attack. At night, I like to have a mint tea like peppermint. A cup of tea is nice to have at night even if I don't want to drink much of it. Just holding the warm mug and taking a few sips are very relaxing.

I try not to snack at all in the evening—not even a fruit snack. I feel better, and I'm less vulnerable to other types of snacking if I just stick with the milk and tea. Eating decisions pursue us to the very end of the day. Everything is going well, the eating day has been successful, and then you hear a family member popping popcorn ...

Occasionally, I have a night meeting in which a specially prepared dessert is served. In a small group, it's hard to turn down a dessert that someone has carefully made for the occasion. Moreover, I sometimes don't *want* to say no. In that case, I skip all beverages with the exception of ice water. If the group is large, or the snack is self-serve, I might more easily forgo the treat. For those times when you want to turn down an evening dessert, it's good to have a few graceful excuses, all of which could very well be true: "It looks so delicious, but I have trouble sleeping if I eat at night"; "I'd love to have some, but I'm still very full from supper"; or "It looks wonderful, but I'm really just thirsty." I hate to make a scene when turning down food. After trying to lose weight for so many years, I'll do anything to avoid calling attention to myself—and my current diet.

Then there is the challenge of the evening party. Most over-eaters try to save calories so they can indulge at the party. But even planned indulgence inevitably leads to more. Soon you'll feel as if you're chained to the snack table. I feel safest when I settle back with a beverage, away from the snacks. Later, I might have a small plate of the homemade or special snacks, skipping the usual, commercially available snacks. Then I settle back once again with some ice water to end consumption.

Many times, I've found myself snacking to stay awake at night. Although I consider myself a morning person, I also like the quiet freedom of the late night hours. When I realize what I'm doing, I need to just walk away from that temptation and go to bed. Getting plenty of sleep is a great help in the normal-izing of eating patterns.

A supporting strategy to end meals

The reliance on easy-to-manage foods, along with reduced con-sumption of difficult-to-manage foods, is the main strategy to decrease overall food consumption in a natural way. However, you may find that you need a supporting strategy in determin-ing how much to eat at a meal. We don't always have control about what we have to eat, especially at suppertime. What is served may be quite difficult-to-manage.

The best way I found to cut back is to establish a simple rule. Eat a moderate plate or bowl of food, wait for a bit, then take a smaller helping of seconds. Waiting before taking seconds increases the length of the meal and may assist you with fullness discernment. I call this the three-point rule: take a moderate helping … wait … then take a smaller second helping.

If you have no control over serving size, such as in a restaurant, you need to reject the notion that you must clean your plate. That was for the days of food scarcity. We live in the days of enormous all-you-can-eat buffets. In table-service restaurants, the servings are oversized and, unfortunately, we eat what we are served.

Devote a few days to consciously cutting back on the amount you would normally consume. During the first day or two, you will miss having big helpings of food. Soon, lesser helpings will feel normal. After you intentionally limit the size of your meals for a few days, your stomach will adjust itself. Your fullness discernment will become more sensitive. If you're afraid you haven't eaten enough and you'll be hungry in an hour, rest assured there are always beverages to drink between meals. Fruits and easy dairy may also be consumed. The easy dairy, in particular, can get you over a rough spot. If such items don't seem appealing, then you'll know you aren't truly hungry.

This rule, along with the other strategies I've mentioned, will help you become more aware of fullness. In summary: Don't drink water before meals to fill up before eating. Whenever possible, rely on easy foods and reduce consumption of difficult foods. Eat a moderate helping of food, wait, and then take a smaller second helping. Finally—a special note to the nibblers among us, like me—don't start picking at leftover food after the meal has ended.

It's vitally important not to eat too much during meals. The more you overeat at mealtimes, the more likely you'll turn to snack food later to relieve the discomfort.

Weight loss

Although the *Four Habits for Normal Eating* do not constitute a weight loss regimen, weight reduction may well occur as a natural consequence. As you follow this plan, your weight will stabilize, and it's likely you'll experience slow but sure weight loss as food cravings diminish and food consumption gradually decreases. Truly, the best advice I can offer is: Keep practicing the four habits. Get better at them, day by day. Be persistent. Be honest with yourself. Allow these habits to fully form.

Despite the call for patience, I know that overeaters are intensely interested in dramatic weight loss. We see the advertisements that promise amazing results in a few weeks of dieting, and we want that too. It is so exciting to see the scale drop five pounds in one week, even if we know most of it is water loss rather than actual fat reduction. The promise of accelerated weight loss is very alluring.

The most logical way to accelerate weight loss is to add an exercise program while you keep following the *Four Habits for Normal Eating*. If you have become discouraged with exercise as a weight loss strategy, it may be time to give it another try. When eating has normalized, an exercise program can have the impact for weight reduction that it is designed for. After consulting with your doctor, find an exercise program that you enjoy and one that fits as seamlessly as possible into your daily schedule. A fitness professional can help you find a program that is suitable and effective.

Diet and exercise are the twin pillars of weight loss. I must admit I was far more interested in diet as a weight loss method. Therefore, I imposed a dieting technique onto my meal guide in the hope of accelerating weight loss. Without going into detail, I tried assigning simple calorie counts to meals in order to decrease food intake. I also limited each beverage or snack to an approximate count of one hundred calories. But I soon chafed under these calorie restrictions, especially at suppertime.

Although I no longer try to lose weight by this method, the calorie analysis and portion adjustments were instructive. I continue to use the calorie-counted portions of my usual breakfast and lunch. I like to be gently mindful of portion sizes because they tend to creep upward over time.

My favorite way to accelerate weight loss consists of eating only easy-to-manage foods for a period of two weeks. During this time, my consumption is naturally suppressed because the taste stimulation of difficult-to-manage foods is absent. When using this method, I eat my usual breakfast, but lunch consists of a generous garden salad sprinkled with garbanzo beans and oil dressing. Supper choices may include Chinese vegetable stir-fry, Mexican beans and rice, and vegan dishes such as ratatouille over rice. Soups may include cream of tomato, split pea, or lentil. I like to stir-fry non-silken tofu to substitute for the filet in the divided plate meal. Tangy foods, such as pickles, cut the monotony of the whole starches and vegetables. I continue to drink juice beverages between meals and eat snacks of fruit and easy dairy. The practice of eating only easy-to-manage foods is challenging—albeit some may say intolerable—because it pulls you out of the mainstream of eating choices. I like this method because the food choices are clear, with no arbitrary restrictions on amount. When I do this, I feel like I'm in boot camp for normal eating. Upon returning to the original plan, I am more skillful at emphasizing easy-to-manage foods.

If you are curious about new diet plans, I think it's fine to try any doctor-approved diet that intrigues you. Then return to normal eating for weight maintenance. There are many diet strategies out there, and they will work well if you are highly motivated. Interesting new ideas are being developed all the time. Rest assured, you can fall back on the *Four Habits for Nor-*

mal Eating when you've reached your goal or when the wave of enthusiasm is spent.

It's OK to ride a wave of weight loss enthusiasm, but know when the wave has reached the shore. Strong motivation comes along once in a while. When the power dissipates, that's when the cheating and even binging start. We all know how quickly pounds can come back on. We thrash around in desperation to renew the power of enthusiasm—but to no avail. When you feel yourself floundering, quickly return to a sure, steady plan for normal eating. This will prevent you from regaining the weight you lost during that time of high motivation.

A time of accelerated weight loss can be a glorious time of success, but it carries hidden dangers. Any concerted effort to lose weight can resurrect old resentments and feelings of self-denial. It may cause you to focus solely on pounds lost rather than the acquirement of normal eating behaviors. A weight loss strategy can invite more than the usual amount of inner conflict during the day, causing you to clutch the problem more closely. Instead, we need to loosen our grip on the problem and move forward into life.

◆   ◆   ◆

Move forward into life

Effective habits for normal eating allow you to relax and move forward into life. As you move forward, the conflicts of temptation gradually drop away. Turn your gaze outward rather than inward. Forget yourself and temptation as you work to make life better, especially for the good of others. Even your daily tasks can be done in this spirit of service. There will be much more about this in Part Four.

When you are trying to eat normally, worries about weight loss may attempt to invade. Don't entertain those worried thoughts. They only stall your forward momentum. There will be times of failure but don't allow those feelings of doubt and discouragement to take root. Set aside some time each day to rest in complete dependence on God. Then prayerfully express your desire to eat normally and lose weight. Summon your faith as you wholeheartedly dedicate yourself to God's will. Then, step forward into the joys of life.

In all this discussion of physical causes and eating strategies, we easily forget the spiritual aspect of this struggle. The *Four Habits for Normal Eating* are very helpful, but these habits are not powerful on their own. Real power for self-change comes through spiritual transformation. Let's go back over some of the points made in the earlier parts of this book. I'd like to reiterate what I said about happiness and then present the *Four Practices for Transcending Everyday Temptations*. This can serve as a daily reminder and a quick review of Parts One through Three, and a preview of Part Four.

Four practices for transcending everyday temptations

Overeaters, like everyone else, are searching for happiness. Food has become the primary way we try to control our own happiness. We eat to induce basic feelings of security, relaxation, stimulation, and pleasure. These four states of well-being can be further understood if elevated to the spiritual emotions of love, peace, hope, and joy.

There is no need to control your happiness with food. There is a better way, a way of spiritual transformation, which leads to happiness. Dependence on God provides the trustworthy love we seek. Wholehearted desire for God's will and presence gives rise to the inner peace we crave. As we deploy faith along with effort, we are filled with the hope that we can achieve our goals. And finally, the joy of living is truly ours as we dare to love and to serve.

As we receive the blessing of happiness through spiritual transformation, we also achieve self-mastery and freedom from temptation. The following four practices can serve as a prayerful reminder of what transcending temptation is all about.

Four Practices
for
Transcending Everyday Temptations

From Part I

Pause to rest a while with God. Lean on him with childlike trust. It's safe to confess your fears and failures. Relinquish control over happiness. Depend on God, rather than **temptation**, for wholeness and security.

From Part II

In prayer, express your desire to eat normally. Offer all your desires and problems to God. Then let go and let God in. Above all, desire God's will and presence. In the liberating light of God's will, **temptations** fade and higher desires flourish.

From Part III

Prepare to do your part to carry out your decisions. Deploy faith along with effort. Through living faith, rely on the trans-forming power of the Spirit. Be assured God will strengthen and guide you through the *temptations* of today.

A preview of Part IV

Resume your duties and join the pursuits of truth, beauty, and goodness. Venture forth, forgetting yourself, as you dare to love and to serve. Pause to give thanks and praise. Be cleansed of *temptation* as you walk the path of life with God.

I.   Depend on God
II. Desire God's will and presence
III. Deploy faith along with effort
IV. Dare to love and to serve

◆   ◆   ◆

Now it is on to Part Four. Do not skip this! The time of planning, as well as prayer, is over. Stand upright in faith and step forward with God.

Let them thank the Lord for his steadfast love,
for his wonderful works to humankind.
For he satisfies the thirsty,
and the hungry he fills with good things.

Psalm 107:8,9

Part 4
You can be set free

There is one more practice in the quest to transcend temptation. It gives meaning and purpose to our lives. The promise of
happiness is fulfilled beyond measure.

Step forward with God

Start saying yes to the noble urgings of life. Step forward with
God. Reenter the world with a clearer head and fresh perspective. There are obligations to meet and schedules to keep. Follow the flow of work and focus on what needs to be done. Start
small and complete what you can. Sprinkle your day with
humor and play. Be friendly with the people around you.

We are privileged to be partners with God in all that we do.
Think with God as you go about your day. It feels good to
know we don't have to work alone. Continue to ask for help
whenever you need it. You're going to need that mysterious
counsel and renewed strength. After making your own way

through life for so long, it's a relief to have a wise and reliable friend with whom to talk things over.

Keep moving on the path of life. We progress along the path through the decisions we make and the actions we take. As we walk through life with God, we learn to make decisions based upon love, and we learn to do his gracious will. Yet, even when we mean well, we will make plenty of mistakes along the way. Don't let that get you down. With God, you can traverse safely through the challenges that lie ahead.

There are plenty of challenges to be encountered in the everyday world of work, play, and relationships. Our ordinary, recurring difficulties in these three realms can greatly exacerbate the temptation to overeat. For example, many of us avoid work by looking in the refrigerator or peering into the snack cupboard. We also misuse our well-earned breaks by grabbing a bag of chips, munching mindlessly with glazed eyes. When troubles rock our relationships, we search out comfort food. Life is full of such difficulties born of habitual and emotional responses. You may need to devote some of your prayer time to this. Offer these persistent problems to God and let in his wisdom and presence. Have faith that he will shine a light on the right place to begin solving them.

Apply some effort to the establishment of better habits about work, play, and relationships. You may have to rework your daily routine so that it suits your energy levels that predictably ebb and flow throughout the day. It's likely you'll need to find satisfying ways to relax besides watching television with a snack by your side. You may need to recognize and improve the typical ways you interact with people. Sometimes this involves refusing to accept the injurious ways other people may treat you. Effective habits regarding work, play, and relationships lessen daily stress and the tendency to engage in temptation. Best of all, good habits allow you to forget yourself and become fully engaged in life.

Our steps are made firm by the Lord,
when he delights in our way;
though we stumble, we shall not fall headlong,
for the Lord holds us by the hand.

Psalm 37:23–24

Forget yourself

The best experiences of life happen when we forget about ourselves. Immerse yourself in the work at hand. Give your complete attention to the person you're with. Allow yourself to relax and fully enjoy a time of play. Slip into the flow of life. Self-consciousness is a distraction from the joy of immediate experience.

For our own sake, we need to forget about ourselves. The self should be like the ring on our finger. It is always there, but we forget about it. When we lose our *self*, it's not that we no longer have a self-identity. What we lose is our self-consciousness. The more we forget about ourselves, the more genuinely real we become.

The less self-conscious we are, the less concerned we'll be about protecting ourselves from failure or from what others might say. It becomes so much easier to make good decisions when we are not trying to embellish or protect the self. Decreasing self-consciousness reduces our vulnerability to fear and its debilitating effects. The less importance we place upon ourselves, the more we are able to make significant contributions through our work. It is wonderful to be freed from the constraints of self-consciousness and self-importance.

When we are God-conscious, that overwhelming sense of self begins to disappear. The self and temptation go hand in hand. It is the self that clamors for the objects of temptation. As the self recedes into the background within the presence of God, temptations recede as well.

> *But let all those that put their trust in thee rejoice:*
> *let them ever shout for joy ...*

> Psalm 5:11a (KJV)

Escape from self-involvement

The problem is, we've become increasingly self-involved as we've struggled with overeating and weight gain. We worry about what the scale is going to say the next time we step on it. We nervously glance at ourselves in the mirror or in the reflecting glass of shop windows as we pass by. We spend a lot of mental energy monitoring our behavior around food. We've been told to keep food diaries, to examine what we eat, how much, when, and speculate as to why. Although this advice can help us be more honest with ourselves, it sure doesn't help us become more self-forgetting. Some self-understanding is helpful, but it can easily become excessive self-examination.

We've become more and more distracted by the techniques of dieting. We count calories and carefully measure our food. We read labels and calculate the fat grams or carbohydrates per serving. We search the latest magazine articles and watch infomercials to learn about a new breakthrough method of weight loss. These distractions have taken us away from full involvement in the world around us.

We also fall into self-absorbed thoughts about future weight loss. We calculate how many weeks it will be before we reach our goal weight. Then, we daydream about the shopping trip for smaller clothes. Even worse, all this thinking about weight loss encourages us to indulge pride. We imagine others admiring us. We fantasize about the glorious days ahead when we'll surprise everyone with our accomplishment and new body. When we're on a roll, we might even indulge self-righteousness, looking down with mild disdain upon others who are still sinking in the mire of this complex problem.

All this self-preoccupation is exhausting. How many people are accomplishing far less than they can because this problem takes up so much of their time and energy? How many relationships haven't started because we're too involved with our own problems? How many adventures have been shelved, waiting for the day when we'll look and feel better about ourselves?

Selfishness is both a cause and effect of the problem of temptation. When I originally defined temptation, I alluded to the idea of selfishness. We are led into temptation by ordinary human selfishness as well as natural tendencies. I raise the idea of selfishness carefully. Overeaters are not more selfish than other people. It may not even occur to us that we're being selfish because we feel more like victims, of tendencies beyond our control, than like selfish perpetrators. Nonetheless, it's in there.

Any time we seek to receive for ourselves, there is an element of selfishness in the motive. This even happens when we try to find happiness in healthier ways. We need to take care of ourselves, yes, but excessive concern for ourselves easily becomes selfishness. Selfishness is the insatiable seeking to receive for oneself. Moreover, the effort to secure happiness is futile. The more we try to capture it, the more it eludes us. The promise of happiness is real, but we need to break out of the tight circle of self in order to realize that promise.

> *Turn my eyes from looking at vanities;*
> *give me life in your ways.*

Psalm 119:37

Refocus your energy

Arrest the energy you previously used in self-seeking behavior and channel it into the work at hand, the other person, or healthy play. Right now, you probably feel most comfortable in one of these three arenas of life. Try venturing into the arena that is least familiar to you. A well-rounded person can enjoy and appreciate their work, some type of play, and a variety of relationships. At every transition during the day, choose the path of life rather than the dead end of temptation. Focus your energy into constructive work, renewing play, and healthy relationships rather than squandering your energy on fighting a losing battle with temptation.

Even when overeating temptations are the greatest, there are ways to redirect your energy. Do you overeat at parties? If you do, turn your attention to the possibilities for play, relationships, and even work at the party. Choose the active option by playing the game or help with the refreshments. Enjoy the conversation and humor. Rather than circling the food table, sit in one spot with a beverage and get to know someone a little better. If you leave a chair open next to you, someone who needs your companionship just may sit down next to you. If you don't feel like talking, do some people-watching. Admire their good qualities and give thanks for them.

Life is bursting with possibilities for participation in truth and beauty, as well as goodness. Join in the pursuits of truth, the creations of beauty, and the expressions of goodness. These divine realities can permeate even the commonplace duties of the day. Being mindful of these higher goals can add a meaningful dimension to all we do.

Ordinary activities can be further uplifted when love is your motive. Through love, your work is elevated to a new level—the level of devoted service. Through love, we desire to do good for others.

Make me to know your ways, O Lord;
teach me your paths.

Psalm 25:4

Dare to love and to serve

In partnership with God, life takes on a feeling of adventure. There are great things to be done even in the seemingly small but magnificently unselfish things we do. Dare to love and to serve. Remember that service takes many forms. Don't get stuck in the rut that says service is just this set of tasks. God provides us with many and various ways to serve that suit the type of person we are and what our talents are.

Ask yourself each day, "What can I do today to make life better for others?" Often, we need search no further than to carry out our everyday duties. Somebody needs to perform the mundane tasks of life. Cheerfully do the ordinary tasks that make life more pleasant for everyone.

Seek to be a blessing to others. Be watchful for things you can do to help. The golden rule of friendly relations gives us a clue to what other people may want and need. Put yourself in their shoes to discover what they long to hear or what they'd appreciate having done for them. Show an interest in them. Give of yourself freely, with no strings attached. Give without thought of receiving in return.

If you're not sure what you can do for someone, saying a prayer for them is often a first step in service. We may not know what is within our capacity to do or give. Prayer heightens our consciousness of the needs of others. Generosity blossoms within us as we pray unselfishly. Praying for others is a good way to develop understanding and love for other people.

In service, we become the living channels for the goodness and love of God. When we do good to others, we are allowing God to love through us. The more we love others, the more we are able to experience God's love because it is passing through us. And the more we live in God's love, the more desire and energy we have to serve others.

Trust in the Lord,
and do good ...

Psalm 37:3a

Rejuvenate with gratitude

Take time each day for gratitude. Just say thank you to God and keep on saying it. If you want to be specific, there is so much to be thankful for. Thank God for comforting you and leading you. Give thanks for family, friends, and the goodness of other people. Express appreciation for the beauty of nature and adventure of living. Allow your words of thanks to become words of praise and adoration. Enter into the joy of worship.

You may be puzzled by the word "worship." In our secular age, it seems like something appropriate only for ancient people who prostrate themselves before the idol of a demanding god. But worship is alive and well in these rational times. Think of how people flock to see a famous person. We go because we want to be near that person, and the experience of adoring that person seems well worth the trouble. Think of how crowds react to the musicians during rock concerts. Our celebrity-crazed culture is a form of misplaced worship. The desire to worship seems to be built into us. If we don't worship God, we will find someone or something else to worship.

The unrecognized spiritual longing to worship can cause us to lapse unwittingly into temptation. A spiritually growing person will begin to experience urges to worship. If we don't recognize this longing for what it really is, we may reach for food in the vain attempt to satisfy this unnamed need. Just as we fell into temptation when we needed to play, we may be intercepted by temptation when we need to worship. Worship provides a deep satisfaction that all our pleasure-seeking activities cannot possibly give.

Allow your soul to be satisfied with the inspiration of true worship. It is something you come to long for once you've experienced it. It is restful, yet stimulating. It is fulfilling and inspiring. Worship is good for us. It helps us to know God and become more like him. It refreshes and rejuvenates us. Worship is an intimate and joyful experience with God.

Freely give your adoration to God. We give our love and adoration to God without thought of receiving, yet in fact we do receive. In worship, we are forgetting about ourselves while standing in awe of the magnificence of God. Worship asks nothing and places no expectations upon God. Be receptive and inviting to the presence of God. Occasionally, you may feel swept up in a mountaintop experience; but do not expect that to happen. A subtle, quiet communion with God is refreshing and stabilizing.

Sometimes worship arises spontaneously. Music can bring on a thankful feeling. The beauty of nature often elicits a feeling of awe for God's universe. A realization of truth can move us to reverence. The relaxation of meditation is useful in the practice of regular worship. The availability of group worship is a great blessing. Be aware, however, that perfunctorily going through an order of worship is not worship; neither is the encouragement of extreme emotion. The design and content of many services of worship so often keep us at arm's length from God. Performance can easily get in the way of worship. Look for communities of worship led by a socially mature and spiritually inspired person. The music and ritual should lead you into a real and satisfying experience with God.

Worship and service are essential in the religious life. If you try to serve without worshipping, you will gradually burn out. If you worship without serving, you'll wonder why worship has become less and less satisfying. True worship of God inspires us to serve our fellows. Conversely, loving service makes us long for communion with God in worship. Worship is like breathing in, and service is like breathing out. We receive the Heavenly Father's love in worship and pour it forth in service to our brothers and sisters here on earth.

As a deer longs for flowing streams,
so my soul longs for you, O God.

My soul thirsts for God, for the living God.
When shall I come and behold the face of God?

Psalm 42:1–2

The path of life

Recommit yourself each day to walking the path of life with God. If you question whether you're on the path, ask yourself two questions: Am I trying to love and honor God? Am I trying to love and serve other people? If we love God, we open our lives to him. If we love other people, we find ways to make life better for them. When we walk this path, we become immersed in a great flow of love. We know we are headed in the right direction.

Gradually it becomes easier to cleanse ourselves of temptation as we daily walk this path. Slowly but surely, the conflicts of temptation drop away. This is the positive approach. We are doing something rather than suppressing something. No longer is it a chore to rid ourselves of a stubborn temptation. No longer is it a bothersome task to change, but a great privilege. There is purifying power in our sincere, spiritual devotion. We are conquering temptation through the love of a higher and better way of life.

As we walk this path, we find the happiness that we have long sought. Love, peace, hope, and joy become ours through wholeheartedly embracing the way of God. Life is filled with meaning and purpose. We begin to experience true freedom and genuine self-mastery. This is the reliable path, which God provides. It is the path of spiritual transformation, which allows us to transcend temptation.

You show me the path of life.
In your presence there is fullness of joy;
in your right hand are pleasures forevermore.

Psalm 16:11

APPENDIX A

Daily Reminders

Now that you have reached the end, I've gathered the various guides into one spot for easy reference. Adapt them and revise them to suit your needs. For example, you may alter the spiritual practices to speak more directly to your own religious tradition. The *Four Practices for Transcending Everyday Temptations* and the *Four Habits for Normal Eating* are designed to help, not to constrain.

Take a bit of time, each day, to read the *Four Practices for Transcending Everyday Temptations,* which can serve as a prayer guide. The essence of the four practices may be easily memorized as a series of four words beginning with the letter D: depend on God, desire God's will and presence, deploy faith along with effort, and dare to love and to serve. As you become more familiar with the *Four Practices*, you won't need thorough, daily review. The phrases beginning with the letter D may be the only reminder you need.

If time allows, it is refreshing to pause between practices two and three to engage in a longer period of meditation or worshipful communion with God. I've found this sequence to be a helpful framework for a satisfying prayer experience. When I get up from prayer and move forward into life, I feel as if I've at least touched upon the essential principles that lead to a genuine happiness.

The four spiritual emotions—love, peace, hope, and joy—are listed, following the *Four Practices*, in an order that corresponds with Parts One through Four. As you will recall, these emotions are elements of happiness, and happiness is what we seek when we engage in temptation. The basic feelings—security, relaxation, stimulation, and pleasure—are also included in corresponding order. In Appendix B, I have a few more things to say about love, peace, hope, and joy.

Also, each day, review the *Four Habits for Normal Eating* and refer to the associated lists of beverages and foods. Soon, these reminders will become habits. Then, you will no longer need to read them each day. As mentioned before, the *Four Habits* may be changed to fit your lifestyle, preferences, and special needs. Although these dietary suggestions are natural and nonrestrictive, it is always recommended that you consult with your doctor regarding your own health and nutritional requirements before embarking on this or any other eating plan.

Four Practices
for
Transcending Everyday Temptations

From Part I

Pause to rest a while with God. Lean on him with childlike trust. It's safe to confess your fears and failures. Relinquish control over happiness. Depend on God, rather than **temptation**, for wholeness and security.

From Part II

In prayer, express your desire to eat normally. Offer all your desires and problems to God. Then let go and let God in. Above all, desire his will and presence. In the liberating light of God's will, **temptations** fade and higher desires flourish.

From Part III

Prepare to do your part to carry out your decisions. Deploy faith along with effort. Through living faith, rely on the transforming power of the Spirit. Be assured God will strengthen and guide you through the **temptations** of today.

From Part IV

Resume your duties and join the pursuits of truth, beauty, and goodness. Venture forth, forgetting yourself, as you dare to love and to serve. Pause to give thanks and praise. Be cleansed of **temptation** as you walk the path of life with God.

Abbreviated Four Practices:

I.   Depend on God
II. Desire God's will and presence
III. Deploy faith along with effort
IV. Dare to love and to serve

Searching for happiness:

I.   Love   Security
II. Peace   Relaxation
III. Hope   Stimulation
IV. Joy   Pleasure

Four Habits for Normal Eating

1. **Rely on water and juice beverages between meals**—to redirect taste desires and diminish food cravings that thirst intensifies.

2. **Rely on easy-to-manage foods for meals, and reduce consumption of difficult-to-manage foods**—to improve hunger/fullness recognition and naturally reduce food consumption.

3. **Rely on a simple meal guide**—to cope with the increased choice and availability of food in modern life.

4. **Rely on breath**—to achieve relaxed alertness and decrease stress-induced eating.

Easy-to-manage foods are attractive when you're truly hungry. **Difficult-to-manage foods** are highly attractive even when you're not hungry.

Easy-to-manage foods	Difficult-to-manage foods
Fruits	Meat, Cheese, Eggs
Easy Dairy 4	Creamy Favorites
Vegetables/Oil	Flour Foods
Whole Starches	Snack Foods

*

A Daily Beverage and Meal Guide
Four Habits for Normal Eating

Time of Day	Beverage Path	Meal Guide
Breakfast	Water* Coffee	Fruit, Milk, Oatmeal
Mid-morning	Fruit herb tea Sweet juice	
Lunch		Veggie-filled Sandwich
Mid-afternoon	Tea Tart juice	
Supper	Salty juice	Vegetables and Main Dish Fruit-filled Dessert
Evening	Milk Mint herb tea	

* Fruits and Easy Dairy are recommended for snacks.
* Drink water freely throughout the day.

Summary of Beverages and Foods
Four Habits for Normal Eating

Beverages

Sweet:	Apple juice and blends, grape juice, apricot nectar, hot cider
Tart:	Orange juice, grapefruit juice, lemonade, cranberry cocktail
Salty:	Tomato juice, vegetable juice
Protein:	Milk*, soy milk, yogurt beverage
Water:	Ice water, herbal tea, sparkling water*, (coffee, tea)

Easy-to-manage foods

Fruits:

Fresh or frozen fruit, canned fruit, applesauce, reconstituted dried fruit

Easy Dairy 4:

Milk, yogurt, cottage cheese, sour cream, and their non-dairy equivalents

Vegetables/Oil:

Steamed or sautéed vegetables, salad with dressing, vegetables with dip

Whole Starches:

Potatoes*, beans, grains, rice, cooked cereal

Difficult-to-manage foods

Meat, Cheese, and Eggs:

Meats including fish, hard and soft cheese, eggs

Creamy Favorites:

Butter—and other spreads such as margarine, mayonnaise, cream cheese, cheese spread, peanut butter

Ice cream—and other desserts such as frozen yogurt, frozen custard, pudding

Whipped cream—and other toppings such as whipped topping, marshmallow

Flour Foods:

Cakes, pastries, cookies, bars

Donuts, coffee cake, croissants, muffins, scones, nut breads

French toast, biscuits, waffles, pancakes, ready-to-eat cereal

Pasta, noodles, dumplings, batter-dipped foods

Breads, bagels, rolls, pita, tortillas, crisp bread

Snack Foods:

Chips, pretzels, crackers, popcorn, puffed snacks

Candy: chocolate, caramel, butterscotch, fruit-flavored, licorice

Snack meats and cheeses, peanuts, nuts

Trail mix, granola bars, soy nuts, sunflower seeds, dried fruit

*Exceptions: Sweetened milk, soft drinks, and high fat preparations of potatoes or other whole starches are difficult-to-manage choices.

APPENDIX B

Selected References

Psalms and Proverbs—Quotations

All quotations from Psalms and Proverbs are from the New Revised Standard Version Bible, with the exception of two quotations from the King James Version (KJV). The passage from Romans in the following paragraph is also from the New Revised Standard Version Bible.

The New Testament—References

There are many significant New Testament passages that inspire the principles in this book. I've chosen to list only passages from the four gospels that may be directly linked to Jesus' use of the phrase "kingdom of heaven" or "kingdom of God." There are different meanings attached to the kingdom concept, but the one I used was set forth by the Apostle Paul when he said in Romans 14:17, "For the kingdom of God is not food and drink but righteousness and peace and joy in the Holy Spirit." In this context, the kingdom of heaven may be thought of as a new and transformed way of living. As this kingdom grows within us, we are increasingly able to transcend temptation and realize the spiritual promises that Jesus proclaimed.

Part I   Depend on God

Matthew 18:1–5	Become like children
Matthew 19:23–26	Hard for a rich person to enter
Matthew 5:3–5	The Beatitudes—first three
Matthew 6:25–34	Do not worry—Strive first for the kingdom

Part II   Desire God's will and presence

Matthew 6:9–15	Your will be done
Matthew 5:6–8	The Beatitudes—fourth and sixth
Luke 17:20–21	The kingdom of God is within you (KJV)
Matthew 13:1–23	The parable of the sower

Part III   Deploy faith along with effort

Matthew 13:33	The parable of the yeast
Matthew 13:31–32	The parable of the mustard seed (see also Luke 17:5–6)
John 3:1–10	You must be born from above
Matthew 13:44–46	Treasure hidden in a field—Pearl of great value

Part IV   Dare to love and to serve

Luke 10:25–37	What must I do to inherit eternal life?
Luke 4:16–21	The Spirit of the Lord is upon me
Matthew 5:7, 9–11	The Beatitudes—fifth, seventh, eighth, ninth
Mark 8:34–35	If any want to become my followers

Love, Peace, Hope, and Joy—I was surprised to discover that the four spiritual emotions of happiness, spoken of in Part I of this book, corresponded to the names that are sometimes given to the four candles in the Christian Advent wreath. The candles are lit in the following order: Hope, Peace, Joy, and Love. After this discovery, I became thoroughly delighted with this foursome. Try matching them to the four seasons of the year and even to the four-part progression of the day: sunrise, daytime, sunset, and nighttime.

The Urantia Book—References

The Urantia Book was of great assistance to me in identifying and sorting the spiritual concepts that are presented in this book. It provided a consistent vision of the fatherly nature of God and of human brotherhood. It helped me to understand the effectiveness of faith and the importance of wholehearted desire to do God's will. Among many fascinating passages, the following were particularly inspirational and useful to me in this endeavor:

Jesus' Teaching at Tyre	Paper 156	Section 5 Paragraphs 3, 4, 5
Lesson on Self-Mastery	Paper 143	Section 2
Sermon on the Kingdom	Paper 137	Section 8
The Young Man Who was Afraid	Paper 130	Section 6
The Consecration of Choice	Paper 111	Section 5
Conditions of Effective Prayer	Paper 91	Section 9
The Universal Father	Paper 1	Introductory section

The Urantia Book was originally published in 1955 by Urantia Foundation. It continues to be published by Urantia Foundation and also by Uversa Press.

Urantia Foundation. *The Urantia Book*. Chicago, IL: Urantia Foundation, 1955.

Uversa Press. *The Urantia Book: Indexed Version*. New York, NY: Uversa Press, 2002.

Buddhism—Quotation

My knowledge about Eastern religions is not extensive enough to attempt many references. However, I came across a passage from Buddhism that stayed with me and helped me. I intentionally recalled this passage whenever I started worrying about weight loss or whenever I thought I should clamp down harder by dieting.

> "How, dear sir, did you cross the flood?" "By not halting friend, and by not straining I crossed the flood." "But how is it, dear sir, that by not halting and by not straining you crossed the flood?" "When I came to a standstill, friend, then I sank; but when I struggled, then I got swept away. It is in this way, friend, that by not halting and by not straining I crossed the flood."

Copyright Bhikkhu Bodhi 2004. Reprinted from *The Connected Discourses of the Buddha* with permission of Wisdom Publications, 199 Elm St., Somerville, MA, 02144, USA.

The Twelve Steps—References

I cannot end this book without paying tribute to the incomparable contribution of the Twelve-Step programs. I have never been a member of Overeaters Anonymous, but for years, I kept close at hand a booklet called *A Guide to the Twelve Steps of Alcoholics Anonymous.* This booklet contains a condensed form of the Twelve Steps that I found very interesting. On pages 1 and 2 of the booklet it says,

The condensed form:

1. We honestly admitted we were powerless over (food) and sincerely wanted to do something about it ...

2. We asked and received help from a power greater than ourselves and another human ...

3. We cleaned up our lives, paid our debts, righted wrongs ...

4. We carried our new way of life to others desperately in need of it ...

This condensed form of the Twelve Steps is similar in sequence to the *Four Practices for Transcending Everyday Temptations,* which, in abbreviated form, are:

I.   Depend on God
II. Desire God's will and presence
III. Deploy faith along with effort
IV. Dare to love and to serve

The Twelve-Step booklet, named above, contains many inspirational thoughts that relate to Parts I–IV of *Transcending the Everyday Temptations of Overeating.* Here is a sampling of quotes:

Relating to Part I:

> "Remember that you are completely dependent on God as you understand Him." (p. 16)

> "Humility is based on the recognition that we are the children of God. It is the consciousness of the need of a power greater than our own and a willingness to let that power control our lives." (p. 9)

Relating to Part II:

> "Instead of asking for outright help, ask for guidance. Ask merely to be shown the way, so that you can do your own part." (p. 9)

> "Make your talks with your Guiding Power a personal thing. Give thanks for help and ask for assistance as though you were addressing your earthly father. Your sincerity is what counts, not the form of language you use." (pp. 13–14)

Relating to Part III:

> "When you meditate on this new way of living you cannot but realize that there is a God above, guiding you through each successive day and night." (p. 13)

> "Very simply put, humility is teachability, an open mind to the truth." (p. 9)

Relating to Part IV:

> "When we help a fellow being, when we are kind to one another we are performing a completely spiritual act. Spiri-

tuality is simply the act of being selflessly helpful. If you will start with this simple explanation you will find that the green light has been flashed on. Christ taught that there are two great commandments: to love God; and to love your neighbor as yourself. If you can follow these you will have no trouble." (p. 14)

Alcoholics Anonymous. *A Guide to the Twelve Steps of Alcoholics Anonymous*. Akron, Ohio: AA of Akron, 1979.

978-0-595-41114-6
0-595-41114-2

Printed in the United States
70576LV00002B/126

9 780595 411146